Independent IBCLC Exam Study Guide 2027-2028:

600 Questions with Detailed Explanations for the International Board Certified Lactation Consultant Exam IBCLC

AF879953

Caldwell Abiodun

Author Introduction

In the earliest days of life, skilled lactation support can profoundly influence both immediate health outcomes and long-term well-being. The International Board Certified Lactation Consultant (IBCLC) exam represents a globally respected standard for healthcare professionals dedicated to advancing breastfeeding care through clinical excellence, ethical practice, and evidence-based knowledge. This study guide has been developed under the direction of an experienced lactation professional who has worked extensively with mothers, infants, and interdisciplinary healthcare teams in diverse clinical settings.

The IBCLC credential, administered by the International Board of Lactation Consultant Examiners (IBLCE), validates advanced competence in lactation management and maternal–infant health. Candidates are assessed across a comprehensive framework that includes development and nutrition, physiology and endocrinology, pathology, pharmacology and toxicology, psychology, sociology and anthropology, as well as techniques and clinical skills. The lead author, in collaboration with a dedicated team of maternal-child health educators, credentialed consultants, and clinical specialists, has carefully structured this guide to align with the current examination blueprint while maintaining practical clinical relevance.

Preparation for the IBCLC examination requires integration of scientific knowledge with critical thinking and compassionate care. This guide moves beyond surface-level review, emphasizing the physiological mechanisms of lactation, infant feeding assessment, management of complex breastfeeding challenges, and safe application of pharmacological principles. Ethical considerations, cultural responsiveness, and effective communication strategies are interwoven throughout the material, reflecting the holistic scope of professional lactation practice.

Recognizing that many IBCLC candidates are practicing healthcare providers balancing demanding schedules, the content is organized for clarity and efficiency. Core concepts are presented in structured sections that build logically, reinforcing both foundational science and applied clinical reasoning. Practice questions are designed to mirror the analytical rigor of the examination, strengthening confidence and promoting mastery rather than rote memorization.

This study guide reflects a deep commitment to advancing standards in lactation consulting. The author and contributing team share a unified goal: to equip candidates with the knowledge, judgment, and confidence necessary not only to succeed on the IBCLC examination, but to provide exceptional, evidence-based care to families during one of the most critical stages of life.

Table of Contents

Author Introduction **2**

Table of Contents **3**

Chapter-1: Development and Nutrition **8**

Infant Feeding Behaviours Across Chronological Stages 8

Term and Preterm Growth and Development 8

Low Birth Weight and Very Low Birth Weight Considerations 9

Infant Nutritional Requirements and Intake Assessment 10

WHO Growth Charts and Gestational Age Adjustment 10

Stooling, Voiding, and Indicators of Adequate Intake 11

Infant Oral Anatomy and Structural Feeding Challenges 11

Complementary Feeding and WHO Introduction Guidelines 12

Milk Banking and Human Milk Sharing 13

Maternal Breast Development, Milk Composition, and Anatomical Variations 13

Chapter-2: Physiology and Endocrinology **14**

Lactogenesis I, II, and III 14

Hormonal Regulation of Milk Production 14

Milk Ejection Reflex and Neuroendocrine Pathways 15

Relactation and Induced Lactation 15

Lactation with Multiples 15

Lactation During Pregnancy and Tandem Feeding 16

Infertility and Assisted Reproductive Technology Considerations 16

Diabetes and Lactation 17

Thyroid, Pituitary, and Polycystic Ovarian Disorders 17

Autoimmune Conditions and Newborn Hypoglycemia 18

Download Audio file and flashcards **19**

Chapter-3: Pathology **20**

Ankyloglossia and Oral Restrictions 20

Cleft Lip, Cleft Palate, and Craniofacial Conditions 20

Congenital and Gastrointestinal Anomalies 20

Gastroesophageal Reflux and GERD 21

Hyperbilirubinemia and Jaundice Management 21
Neurological Disabilities and Feeding Implications 22
Infant Infections and Vertically Transmitted Diseases 22
Maternal Mastitis, Abscess, and Inflammatory Conditions 23
Milk Supply Disorders, Nipple Trauma, and Maternal Systemic Disease 23
Chapter-4 : Pharmacology and Toxicology 24
Alcohol and Lactation 24
Nicotine, Tobacco, and Vaping 24
Cannabis and Breastfeeding 24
Drugs of Abuse and Substance Use Disorders 25
Prescription and Over-the-Counter Medications 25
Labor and Delivery Medications 26
Contraception and Hormonal Influence 26
Galactagogues and Milk Supply Agents 26
Herbs, Supplements, and Alternative Therapies 27
Chemotherapy, Radiation, and Diagnostic Exposures 27
Chapter-5: Psychology, Sociology, and Anthropology 29
Transition to Parenthood and Identity Development 29
Maternal Mental Health and Mood Disorders 29
Cognitive and Psychological Conditions 30
Breastfeeding Dyad Attachment and Bonding 30
Cultural Beliefs and Feeding Practices 30
Family Systems and Support Networks 31
Employment, Workplace Policy, and Lactation 31
Birth Practices and Early Feeding Influence 32
Safe Sleep and Infant Care Practices 32
Weaning Across Developmental Stages 33
Chapter-6: Techniques 34
The First Hour and Early Initiation 34
Skin-to-Skin (Kangaroo Care) 34
Positioning and Hands-Off Techniques 35

Latch Mechanics and Assessment......35
Effective Milk Transfer Evaluation......35
Managing Low Milk Supply......36
Managing Oversupply and Engorgement......36
Medically Indicated Supplementation......37
Milk Expression: Hand Expression and Pumping......37
Breast and Bottle Refusal Management......37
Chapter-7: Clinical Skills......39
Feeding Devices and Alternative Feeding Methods......39
Pumps, Nipple Devices, and Equipment Use......39
Handling and Storage of Human Milk......39
Scale Use and Milk Transfer Measurement......40
Communication Technology and Virtual Care......40
Comprehensive Lactation Assessment......41
Clinical Reasoning and Care Planning......41
Documentation and Professional Communication......41
Interdisciplinary Collaboration and Referral......42
Quality Improvement, Ethics, and Professional Boundaries......42
Chapter 8 – Practice Question and Answers......43
Questions (1-100)......43
Answer key and Explanation (1-100)......54
Questions (101-200)......63
Answer key and Explanation (101-200)......75
Questions (201-300)......83
Answer key and Explanation (201-300)......94
Questions (301-400)......101
Answer key and Explanation (301-400)......112
Questions (401-500)......119
Answer key and Explanation (401-500)......130
Questions (501-600)......138
Answer key and Explanation (501-600)......150

Disclaimer

Chapter-1: Development and Nutrition

Infant Feeding Behaviours Across Chronological Stages

Infant feeding behaviour evolves in predictable stages that correspond to neurological maturity, gestational age, and developmental progression. During the prenatal period, nutritive sucking begins to develop in utero as early as 28 weeks' gestation, with coordination of suck, swallow, and breathe typically maturing between 32 and 34 weeks. Preterm infants may demonstrate immature patterns including weak suction, poor rhythm, and increased fatigue during feeds. Understanding these early patterns is critical when supporting late preterm and very low birth weight infants.

In the first 0–2 days postpartum, feeding behaviour is strongly influenced by birth practices, medication exposure, and early skin-to-skin contact. Healthy term infants typically display a sequence of instinctive behaviours during the first hour, including alertness, rooting, hand-to-mouth activity, and spontaneous latching. Feeding sessions may be brief but frequent. Colostrum volumes are small but physiologically appropriate, and frequent feeding stimulates lactogenesis II.

Between days 3 and 14, feeding becomes more organized. Cluster feeding is common and supports increasing milk supply. Infants begin to show clearer hunger cues such as stirring, rooting, and sucking motions before crying. Crying is a late feeding cue and may interfere with effective latch. Responsive feeding supports optimal milk transfer and supply regulation.

From 1 to 3 months, infants develop improved head control and more efficient sucking patterns. Feeds may become shorter as milk transfer becomes more effective. By 4 to 6 months, distractibility may increase due to neurological development. At approximately 6 months, developmental readiness for complementary feeding includes the ability to sit with support, diminished tongue-thrust reflex, and interest in food.

Between 7 and 12 months, breastfeeding continues to provide significant nutrition and immune protection while solid foods complement intake. Beyond 12 months, breastfeeding remains biologically normal and continues to support emotional regulation, immune function, and nutritional supplementation.

An IBCLC must assess feeding behaviours within the context of gestational age, chronological age, medical conditions, and environmental influences. Recognition of normal variation prevents unnecessary intervention while identifying early signs of dysfunction allows timely support.

Term and Preterm Growth and Development

Growth patterns differ significantly between term and preterm infants, requiring careful interpretation using appropriate growth standards. Term infants are assessed using standard growth charts, whereas preterm infants require gestational age correction until at least two years of age. Failure to correct for prematurity may result in misclassification of growth adequacy.

In the immediate postnatal period, weight loss of up to 7–10 percent in term infants is considered physiologically normal. Excessive weight loss may indicate suboptimal milk transfer or delayed lactogenesis. Preterm infants often experience more complex nutritional challenges due to immature gastrointestinal function, higher metabolic demands, and limited nutrient stores.

Low birth weight and very low birth weight infants require increased protein, calcium, phosphorus, and caloric density to support catch-up growth and neurodevelopment. Human milk provides immunologic protection and improved feeding tolerance; however, fortification may be required in certain clinical contexts to meet elevated nutrient needs.

Growth assessment must include weight, length, and head circumference. Head growth is particularly significant as it reflects brain development. Deviations from expected growth velocity require comprehensive feeding evaluation, including latch effectiveness, feeding frequency, maternal milk supply, and potential medical pathology.

Late preterm infants present unique challenges. Though often similar in size to term infants, they may demonstrate immature feeding coordination, increased sleepiness, and decreased stamina, increasing the risk of inadequate intake. Close monitoring during the first weeks is essential.

An IBCLC integrates growth data with clinical feeding assessment. Growth faltering should prompt evaluation of milk transfer through observation and, when indicated, pre- and post-feed weights. Conversely, rapid weight gain may be associated with over-supplementation or feeding misinterpretation.

Effective lactation support requires understanding the physiologic growth trajectory of both term and preterm infants, recognizing normal patterns, and intervening appropriately when deviations occur.

Low Birth Weight and Very Low Birth Weight Considerations

Low birth weight infants, defined as weighing less than 2500 grams at birth, and very low birth weight infants, weighing less than 1500 grams, present complex lactation management challenges. These infants are often preterm, though some may be growth-restricted at term. Their feeding ability depends on neurologic maturity, cardiorespiratory stability, and gastrointestinal function.

Very low birth weight infants frequently require respiratory support, tube feeding, and careful fluid management in the neonatal intensive care setting. Direct breastfeeding may initially be limited; therefore, early and frequent milk expression is essential to establish maternal supply. Initiation of milk expression within the first hour postpartum significantly improves long-term milk production.

Human milk is particularly protective in this population. It reduces the risk of necrotizing enterocolitis, sepsis, and feeding intolerance. Colostrum provides immunoglobulins and growth factors critical for intestinal maturation. However, due to high nutrient requirements, fortification is often necessary to support adequate growth velocity.

Transition to the breast should occur as soon as the infant demonstrates physiologic readiness. Non-nutritive sucking at the breast during tube feeds can support oral skill development. Kangaroo care enhances physiologic stability, improves milk supply, and facilitates breastfeeding progression.

IBCLCs must collaborate closely with neonatal teams. Monitoring includes weight gain trends, tolerance of feeds, stool patterns, and signs of feeding fatigue. Feeding sessions may need to be shorter and more frequent to prevent energy depletion.

Parental education is crucial. Families may experience anxiety regarding milk sufficiency and infant fragility. Providing clear guidance on pumping schedules, milk storage, and developmental expectations promotes confidence and continuity of breastfeeding after discharge.

Management of low and very low birth weight infants requires advanced knowledge of neonatal physiology, lactation maintenance strategies, and interdisciplinary coordination to optimize outcomes.

Infant Nutritional Requirements and Intake Assessment

Human milk is uniquely adapted to meet the nutritional needs of the human infant. It provides appropriate macronutrient balance, bioavailable micronutrients, immunologic components, enzymes, and bioactive factors. The composition of milk evolves from colostrum to transitional milk to mature milk, adjusting to developmental requirements.

Energy requirements for term infants average approximately 100–120 kcal/kg/day, though needs vary based on gestational age and medical condition. Preterm infants often require higher caloric intake to support catch-up growth. Protein is essential for lean body mass and neurodevelopment, while fats provide critical long-chain polyunsaturated fatty acids for brain and retinal development.

Assessment of adequate intake relies primarily on clinical indicators rather than maternal perception. Indicators include appropriate weight gain, adequate stooling and voiding patterns, audible swallowing during feeds, and infant satisfaction following feeding. In the first week, progression from meconium to transitional stools indicates adequate colostrum intake.

Signs of inadequate intake may include persistent weight loss beyond expected norms, decreased urine output, lethargy, jaundice exacerbation, and poor feeding endurance. Evaluation must consider latch quality, feeding frequency, maternal milk supply, and possible anatomical or neurological concerns.

Responsive feeding supports physiologic intake regulation. Scheduled feeding without regard to cues may impair supply and intake adequacy. IBCLCs must educate families about early hunger cues and normal feeding variability.

Comprehensive intake assessment integrates growth data, feeding observation, maternal history, and infant behaviour. Early identification of feeding challenges prevents complications such as dehydration, hyperbilirubinemia, and failure to thrive.

WHO Growth Charts and Gestational Age Adjustment

Accurate growth assessment is foundational to lactation management. Growth charts provide a standardized method to evaluate infant growth patterns over time. For term infants, standard growth charts are used to monitor weight, length, and head circumference. For preterm infants, gestational age correction must be applied when plotting measurements.

Gestational age adjustment accounts for the number of weeks born before 40 weeks' gestation. Corrected age is calculated by subtracting the number of weeks premature from chronological age. This correction should be used for at least the first two years of life to avoid misinterpretation of developmental and growth progress.

Weight trajectories should follow a consistent percentile channel after the initial postnatal weight loss period. Crossing percentiles downward may signal inadequate intake, while rapid upward shifts may indicate overfeeding or metabolic concerns.

Head circumference is a critical parameter reflecting brain growth. In preterm infants, steady head growth is particularly important and may be influenced by nutritional adequacy.

IBCLCs must understand that growth percentiles represent statistical distribution, not grading scales. An infant in the 10th percentile may be perfectly healthy if following a consistent curve. Parental concern often arises from misunderstanding percentile interpretation.

Clinical assessment should focus on growth velocity rather than single data points. Consistent monitoring and documentation allow early detection of deviations.

Appropriate use of growth charts ensures accurate evaluation, prevents unnecessary supplementation, and supports individualized lactation care plans.

Stooling, Voiding, and Indicators of Adequate Intake

Assessment of stooling and voiding patterns is a fundamental clinical tool for determining adequacy of milk intake in the early weeks of life. In the immediate newborn period, elimination patterns reflect both physiologic transition and feeding effectiveness. During the first 24 hours, at least one void and one meconium stool are expected. Meconium is thick, dark, and tarry, composed of intestinal epithelial cells, lanugo, mucus, and amniotic fluid debris accumulated in utero. Passage of meconium indicates gastrointestinal patency and initial colostrum intake. Over the next several days, stools transition from black meconium to greenish transitional stools and then to mustard-yellow, seedy stools in the breastfed infant, typically by day four or five if intake is adequate. Failure to transition from meconium by day four may suggest insufficient milk transfer and warrants prompt feeding assessment. Urine output also follows a predictable pattern; by day three, at least three wet diapers per day are expected, increasing to six or more by day five. Pale, dilute urine suggests adequate hydration, whereas concentrated urine with urate crystals may indicate insufficient intake. After lactogenesis II, stool frequency in exclusively breastfed infants often ranges from three to eight stools per day in early infancy, although wide variation can be normal once weight gain is established. Some healthy breastfed infants may stool after every feeding, while others may have fewer but soft stools. Hard, pellet-like stools are not typical of exclusively breastfed infants and require evaluation. In addition to elimination patterns, other indicators of adequate intake include audible swallowing during feeds, rhythmic suck-swallow-breathe coordination, visible relaxation after feeding, appropriate weight gain, and sustained alertness. Signs of inadequate intake include persistent sleepiness during feeds, weak suck, decreased urine output, scant or delayed stooling, excessive weight loss, and hyperbilirubinemia. IBCLCs must integrate elimination data with direct feeding observation and growth trends rather than relying on diaper counts alone. Education of families regarding normal variation prevents unnecessary supplementation while ensuring that early signs of suboptimal intake are identified promptly. Careful documentation of stool and urine patterns during the first two weeks provides a noninvasive and highly valuable indicator of breastfeeding effectiveness and neonatal well-being.

Infant Oral Anatomy and Structural Feeding Challenges

Effective breastfeeding depends on coordinated interaction between infant oral structures and maternal breast anatomy. The newborn oral cavity is uniquely adapted for feeding, with a relatively large tongue that fills the oral space, prominent buccal fat pads for stabilization, and a high, soft palate that supports suction generation. During nutritive sucking, the tongue cups around the nipple and areola, creating a seal while peristaltic tongue movements compress the lactiferous sinuses against the hard palate. Jaw excursion contributes to milk removal, and synchronized swallowing protects the airway. Structural variations can disrupt this process and lead to ineffective milk transfer, maternal nipple pain, or poor weight gain. Ankyloglossia, characterized by a restrictive lingual frenulum, may limit tongue elevation or extension, impairing latch depth and tongue mobility. Clinical signs include clicking sounds during feeding, shallow latch, maternal nipple trauma, prolonged feeds, and inadequate weight gain. Assessment must evaluate functional limitation rather than appearance alone. Other oral anomalies such as cleft lip or palate alter intraoral pressure dynamics and may require specialized positioning, pacing techniques, or alternative feeding devices. Micrognathia, retrognathia, and high-arched palate can also interfere with effective latch by altering nipple positioning within the oral cavity. Neurological conditions affecting tone, such as hypotonia or hypertonia, may impair suck-swallow coordination. Late preterm infants frequently demonstrate immature oral motor patterns, leading to fatigue and inconsistent milk transfer. IBCLCs must perform comprehensive oral assessments including observation of tongue movement, palate contour, jaw symmetry, and suck strength. Direct feeding observation is essential to correlate anatomical findings with functional impact. Management may include latch optimization, positioning adjustments, use of breast compressions, oral motor exercises when appropriate, or referral for further evaluation. Early identification and intervention are critical to prevent secondary complications such as low milk supply or early cessation of breastfeeding. A thorough understanding of infant oral anatomy and biomechanics enables the lactation consultant to differentiate between normal variation and clinically significant structural challenges.

Complementary Feeding and WHO Introduction Guidelines

Complementary feeding marks a developmental transition in which solid or semi-solid foods are introduced while breastfeeding continues. Exclusive breastfeeding is recommended for approximately the first six months of life, after which complementary foods are added to meet increasing energy and micronutrient requirements while human milk remains a significant nutritional source. Developmental readiness cues are more reliable than chronological age alone. Indicators of readiness include the ability to sit with minimal support, stable head and neck control, diminished tongue-thrust reflex, coordinated hand-to-mouth movements, and demonstrated interest in food. Introducing solids before developmental readiness may increase choking risk and reduce breast milk intake without nutritional benefit. Human milk continues to provide immune protection, high-quality protein, and essential fatty acids during the complementary feeding period. Iron requirements increase around six months as prenatal iron stores decline; therefore, iron-rich complementary foods such as meats or iron-fortified options are important additions. Complementary feeding should be responsive and paced, allowing the infant to regulate intake while preserving breastfeeding frequency. Breastfeeding should generally precede solid feeds in early introduction stages to maintain milk supply. Cultural feeding practices influence food choices and timing; IBCLCs must provide culturally sensitive guidance while supporting nutritional adequacy. Texture progression is important for oral motor development, transitioning from pureed to mashed to appropriately sized soft finger foods as skills mature. Continued breastfeeding beyond one year remains biologically normal and contributes meaningful nutrition and immunologic protection. Premature discontinuation of breastfeeding during complementary feeding may increase risk of infection and nutritional imbalance. Lactation professionals must educate families that complementary feeding supplements rather than replaces breastfeeding during the first year. Careful counseling prevents misconceptions that solids should rapidly replace breastfeeds and reinforces the role of continued lactation in supporting optimal growth and development throughout infancy.

Milk Banking and Human Milk Sharing

Human milk banking provides pasteurized donor milk for infants who do not have access to their mother's own milk, particularly premature or medically fragile infants. Donor milk is typically prioritized for very low birth weight infants due to its protective effect against necrotizing enterocolitis and other morbidities. Milk banks screen donors through medical history, serologic testing, and lifestyle assessment to minimize infectious risk. Collected milk undergoes pasteurization to eliminate pathogens while retaining many immunologic and nutritional properties. Although some bioactive components are reduced by pasteurization, donor milk remains superior to formula for vulnerable populations. Informal milk sharing, in contrast, occurs outside regulated milk bank systems and carries potential risks including infectious transmission, medication exposure, or contamination. IBCLCs must provide balanced, nonjudgmental education regarding risks and benefits while respecting parental autonomy. Safe handling, storage, and transport of human milk are critical to maintain quality. Families of preterm infants should be counseled on the importance of early and frequent expression to maximize availability of maternal milk, as mother's own milk remains the optimal feeding choice. In situations where maternal milk supply is limited, donor milk may be used as a bridge while lactation support continues. Ethical considerations include equitable access, informed consent, and prioritization policies within neonatal units. Education should clarify that donor milk is not equivalent to maternal milk in terms of immunologic specificity but provides substantial benefits compared with artificial substitutes. IBCLCs play an important advocacy role in promoting systems that increase access to safe donor milk while simultaneously supporting mothers in establishing and maintaining their own milk supply.

Maternal Breast Development, Milk Composition, and Anatomical Variations

Breast development begins in embryonic life and progresses through puberty under hormonal influence. During puberty, estrogen stimulates ductal growth while progesterone supports lobuloalveolar development. Pregnancy induces further mammogenesis through coordinated hormonal activity including estrogen, progesterone, prolactin, and human placental lactogen. Adequate glandular tissue development is necessary for full milk production, though breast size alone does not predict lactation capacity because adipose tissue contributes significantly to volume. Anatomical variations such as widely spaced breasts, significant asymmetry, or tubular breast shape may be associated with insufficient glandular tissue and require careful postpartum monitoring. Nipple structure also varies; protruding nipples facilitate latch but flat or inverted nipples do not preclude successful breastfeeding when appropriate latch techniques are used. Surgical history including reduction, augmentation, or biopsy may impact milk ducts and nerve supply depending on surgical technique. Milk composition evolves dynamically from colostrum, which is rich in immunoglobulins and growth factors, to transitional milk and then mature milk. Foremilk and hindmilk differences reflect fat concentration changes during a feed rather than separate milk types. Human milk contains carbohydrates primarily as lactose, lipids including essential fatty acids, high-quality proteins, enzymes, hormones, and immune components that adapt to the infant's needs. Maternal nutritional status influences certain micronutrient levels but has limited impact on macronutrient composition in well-nourished populations. Endocrine disorders, retained placental fragments, or severe postpartum hemorrhage may interfere with lactogenesis II. IBCLCs must conduct thorough maternal histories including endocrine conditions, prior breast surgery, and anatomical concerns to anticipate potential challenges. Understanding breast physiology and milk composition allows targeted interventions that protect milk supply and optimize breastfeeding outcomes.

Chapter-2: Physiology and Endocrinology

Lactogenesis I, II, and III

Lactogenesis is the process by which the mammary gland develops the capacity to synthesize and secrete milk, and it occurs in three distinct stages regulated by complex hormonal interactions. Lactogenesis I begins approximately midway through pregnancy and continues until birth. During this stage, the mammary epithelium differentiates into secretory cells under the influence of prolactin, estrogen, progesterone, insulin, and cortisol. Colostrum is produced in small quantities, rich in immunoglobulins and bioactive factors. Although prolactin levels are elevated during pregnancy, high circulating progesterone inhibits copious milk secretion by blocking prolactin receptor activity at the alveolar level. Lactogenesis II is triggered by delivery of the placenta, resulting in a rapid decline in progesterone and allowing prolactin to act unopposed on mammary receptors. This stage typically begins between 30 and 72 hours postpartum and is characterized by increased milk volume, commonly described as the onset of copious milk production. Effective and frequent milk removal during this critical window enhances prolactin receptor upregulation and long-term milk supply. Delayed lactogenesis II may occur in association with maternal obesity, diabetes, cesarean birth, retained placental fragments, or severe postpartum hemorrhage. Lactogenesis III, also referred to as galactopoiesis, represents the maintenance phase of milk production and is primarily regulated by autocrine control. Once established, milk synthesis becomes dependent on supply-and-demand mechanisms rather than endocrine dominance. Frequent and effective milk removal maintains production, while milk stasis leads to feedback inhibition through accumulation of local inhibitory peptides within the alveoli. Understanding these stages enables timely identification of disruptions in milk production and supports targeted interventions that protect lactation establishment and long-term maintenance.

Hormonal Regulation of Milk Production

Milk production depends on coordinated endocrine signaling involving prolactin, oxytocin, insulin, cortisol, thyroid hormones, and growth hormone. Prolactin, secreted by the anterior pituitary, is the principal hormone responsible for milk synthesis. Its release is stimulated by nipple stimulation and removal of milk from the breast. Prolactin levels peak during and shortly after feeding, reinforcing continued milk production. Nighttime prolactin surges are particularly significant, making nocturnal feeds important for establishing and sustaining supply. Oxytocin, produced by the hypothalamus and released by the posterior pituitary, mediates milk ejection by causing contraction of myoepithelial cells surrounding the alveoli. Psychological factors strongly influence oxytocin release; stress, pain, and anxiety may inhibit let-down despite adequate milk production. Insulin and cortisol support metabolic processes required for milk synthesis, while thyroid hormones regulate basal metabolic rate and influence lactation efficiency. Hypothyroidism may impair supply, whereas hyperthyroidism may alter maternal metabolic balance. Growth hormone contributes to mammary gland development and functional capacity. Following the early postpartum endocrine-driven phase, local control mechanisms dominate. Accumulation of milk within the alveoli increases intramammary pressure and reduces further synthesis through feedback pathways. Effective milk removal prevents this inhibitory process and maintains production. Endocrine disorders such as pituitary insufficiency, polycystic ovarian syndrome, and diabetes may disrupt hormonal balance and require careful evaluation. A comprehensive understanding of hormonal regulation allows identification of physiologic versus mechanical causes of low supply and guides appropriate management strategies.

Milk Ejection Reflex and Neuroendocrine Pathways

The milk ejection reflex is a neuroendocrine response that facilitates transfer of milk from the alveoli to the nipple. It is initiated by tactile stimulation of the nipple and areola, which activates sensory nerve pathways transmitting signals to the hypothalamus. In response, oxytocin is released from the posterior pituitary into systemic circulation. Oxytocin binds to receptors on myoepithelial cells surrounding the alveoli, causing rhythmic contraction and propulsion of milk through the ductal system toward the nipple. This reflex can occur multiple times during a feeding session and may be experienced subjectively as tingling, pressure, or warmth in the breast, although some individuals perceive no physical sensation. Emotional and psychological states significantly influence oxytocin release. Stress, fear, embarrassment, or acute pain may inhibit the reflex by activating sympathetic pathways that counteract oxytocin's effects. Conversely, relaxation, confidence, and infant cues such as crying or visual contact can trigger conditioned let-down responses even in the absence of direct stimulation. In the early postpartum period, the reflex may be less predictable as neural pathways are still being reinforced through repeated feeding. Over time, consistent stimulation strengthens neuroendocrine responsiveness. Dysfunction of the milk ejection reflex may present as delayed flow, infant frustration at the breast, or maternal reports of poor milk transfer despite adequate supply. Management focuses on optimizing latch, reducing stress, ensuring privacy, and encouraging frequent feeding or pumping to condition reflex pathways. Understanding the neuroendocrine basis of milk ejection underscores the importance of emotional support and environmental factors in successful lactation.

Relactation and Induced Lactation

Relactation refers to the process of reestablishing milk production after a period of partial or complete cessation, whereas induced lactation describes initiation of milk production in individuals who have not experienced recent pregnancy. Both processes rely on stimulating prolactin secretion and promoting mammary gland activation through frequent breast stimulation and milk removal. The fundamental principle is that mechanical stimulation can upregulate prolactin receptors and initiate or restore milk synthesis even in the absence of pregnancy-related hormonal priming, although outcomes vary depending on duration of prior lactation, breast tissue development, and individual endocrine responsiveness. In relactation, success is more likely when some milk production persists and when the interval since weaning is short. Intensive stimulation through nursing, pumping, or hand expression at least eight to twelve times per day is typically required. Skin-to-skin contact enhances oxytocin release and infant interest at the breast. Supplemental feeding methods that allow continued breast stimulation may support transition from artificial feeds to breastfeeding. Induced lactation often requires hormonal preparation to simulate pregnancy, followed by abrupt withdrawal to mimic postpartum hormonal shifts, in addition to mechanical stimulation. Galactagogues may be considered in certain cases, though stimulation remains the primary driver of supply. Emotional support is critical, as the process demands sustained effort and patience. Clear counseling regarding realistic expectations prevents discouragement. Successful relactation or induced lactation demonstrates the adaptability of the human lactation system and highlights the central role of demand-driven physiology in milk production.

Lactation with Multiples

Breastfeeding multiples presents unique physiologic and logistical considerations but is fully compatible with normal lactation capacity. Milk production is governed by demand; therefore, simultaneous feeding of twins or higher-order multiples stimulates increased prolactin receptor activity and greater overall milk synthesis. The mammary gland is capable of adjusting production to meet the needs of more than one infant when effective and frequent milk removal occurs. Early establishment is crucial, particularly if infants are premature or require neonatal support. Initiation of milk expression within the first hour postpartum and maintenance of frequent stimulation protect long-term supply. Feeding strategies may include simultaneous nursing, alternating breasts between infants, or individualized approaches based on infant strength and coordination. Monitoring weight gain for each infant ensures equitable intake. Mothers of multiples may experience increased fatigue, making social and practical support essential. Adequate maternal nutrition and hydration support metabolic demands, though milk composition remains relatively stable across varying maternal intakes in well-nourished populations. Challenges may include delayed lactogenesis associated with preterm birth, increased risk of maternal anemia, and logistical complexity of positioning and scheduling. Education regarding tandem positioning techniques and efficient feeding routines enhances sustainability. With proper support and frequent milk removal, lactation for multiples reflects the same supply-and-demand physiology observed in singleton breastfeeding, demonstrating the remarkable adaptability of the endocrine and autocrine systems governing milk production.

Lactation During Pregnancy and Tandem Feeding

Lactation during pregnancy and tandem feeding involve complex hormonal interactions that influence milk production and composition. During pregnancy, rising levels of estrogen and progesterone promote mammary gland growth while simultaneously inhibiting copious milk secretion. Individuals who conceive while breastfeeding often notice a gradual decline in milk supply during the first or second trimester due to hormonal suppression of prolactin receptor activity. Milk composition may shift toward colostrum in mid-to-late pregnancy, resulting in changes in taste and volume that some nursing children may resist. Despite reduced volume, breastfeeding during an uncomplicated pregnancy is generally safe, as nipple stimulation releases oxytocin in physiologic pulses insufficient to initiate labor in the absence of obstetric risk factors. However, in pregnancies complicated by preterm labor risk, cervical insufficiency, or recurrent miscarriage, individualized clinical guidance is warranted. Tandem feeding after birth requires the mammary gland to respond to the needs of both the newborn and the older child. Colostrum remains available to the newborn despite continued nursing by the older sibling, as colostrum production is hormonally regulated and not depleted by prior feeding. After lactogenesis II, milk production adjusts according to demand from both children. Positioning strategies and clear feeding boundaries may help families manage practical and emotional aspects of tandem feeding. Adequate maternal nutrition, rest, and support are essential, as energy demands increase with concurrent pregnancy and lactation or with feeding multiple children postpartum. Understanding endocrine regulation and maternal physiological capacity allows appropriate counseling that balances safety, maternal well-being, and family preferences.

Infertility and Assisted Reproductive Technology Considerations

Infertility and assisted reproductive technologies may influence lactation through both hormonal and psychological pathways. Conditions such as polycystic ovarian syndrome, hypothalamic dysfunction, and luteal phase abnormalities reflect underlying endocrine imbalances that may affect mammary gland development and prolactin responsiveness. Individuals who conceive through ovulation induction, in vitro fertilization, or other assisted methods may have histories of hormonal treatment that alter baseline endocrine function. Elevated androgen levels in polycystic ovarian syndrome may impair adequate glandular development during puberty and pregnancy, potentially contributing to insufficient milk supply postpartum. Additionally, insulin resistance frequently associated with this condition can interfere with effective lactogenesis II. Individuals with hypothalamic amenorrhea may have altered prolactin dynamics due to stress or energy imbalance. Emotional stress associated with infertility treatment may also affect oxytocin release and early milk ejection reflex responsiveness. Despite these considerations, many individuals with infertility histories breastfeed successfully when provided with early lactation support. Antenatal counseling should include discussion of potential risk factors for delayed lactogenesis, especially in cases involving cesarean birth, multiple gestation, or pregnancy complications. Early initiation of breastfeeding or milk expression, frequent stimulation, and careful monitoring of infant weight gain are protective strategies. A comprehensive endocrine history allows identification of individuals at risk for milk supply challenges and supports proactive management rather than reactive intervention after feeding problems emerge.

Diabetes and Lactation

Diabetes, whether pregestational or gestational, influences lactation physiology through metabolic and hormonal pathways. Insulin plays an important role in mammary gland function by supporting cellular uptake of glucose necessary for lactose synthesis, which drives milk volume through osmotic regulation. Insulin resistance or deficiency may delay lactogenesis II and reduce early milk supply. Individuals with poorly controlled blood glucose during pregnancy are at increased risk of delayed onset of copious milk production. Additionally, infants born to diabetic mothers have a higher incidence of hypoglycemia in the immediate postpartum period due to hyperinsulinemia induced by intrauterine glucose exposure. Early and frequent breastfeeding supports stabilization of neonatal blood glucose and reduces the need for supplementation when milk transfer is effective. Skin-to-skin contact immediately after birth enhances metabolic adaptation and promotes early feeding behaviors. Maternal glycemic control postpartum remains important, as fluctuating glucose levels may affect energy and overall well-being, indirectly influencing feeding frequency and effectiveness. Individuals using insulin should monitor glucose carefully, as breastfeeding can increase caloric expenditure and predispose to hypoglycemia if intake is insufficient. Nutritional counseling emphasizing balanced carbohydrate intake supports both glycemic stability and milk production. With appropriate management, diabetes is not a contraindication to breastfeeding, and lactation may confer long-term metabolic benefits for both parent and child. Understanding the bidirectional relationship between insulin physiology and lactation supports comprehensive care planning in this population.

Thyroid, Pituitary, and Polycystic Ovarian Disorders

Thyroid and pituitary function play essential roles in the regulation of lactation. Thyroid hormones influence basal metabolic rate and cellular energy utilization, both of which affect milk synthesis. Hypothyroidism may present with low milk supply, fatigue, and delayed lactogenesis II, particularly if inadequately treated. Hyperthyroidism may alter metabolic balance and require careful medication management to ensure compatibility with breastfeeding. Screening and appropriate endocrine management are critical when lactation difficulties coexist with systemic symptoms such as weight changes, temperature intolerance, or mood disturbances. Pituitary disorders can have profound effects on lactation. Prolactin deficiency due to pituitary insufficiency impairs milk synthesis, while structural damage to the pituitary from severe postpartum hemorrhage may result in failure of lactogenesis. In contrast, prolactin-secreting adenomas may elevate baseline prolactin levels but do not necessarily guarantee adequate milk production, as receptor responsiveness and milk removal remain critical. Polycystic ovarian syndrome involves complex interactions between insulin resistance, hyperandrogenism, and ovarian dysfunction. Elevated androgens may impair breast tissue development and reduce prolactin receptor sensitivity. Individuals with this condition may experience insufficient glandular tissue or delayed milk production. Early lactation assessment, frequent feeding or pumping, and metabolic optimization improve outcomes. Recognition of endocrine disorders as underlying contributors to supply challenges prevents misattribution to technique alone and allows coordinated medical management that supports sustained lactation.

Autoimmune Conditions and Newborn Hypoglycemia

Autoimmune disorders encompass a wide range of conditions that may affect lactation directly or indirectly through systemic inflammation and endocrine disruption. Conditions such as type 1 diabetes, autoimmune thyroid disease, and systemic inflammatory disorders may influence hormonal balance and energy metabolism, potentially impacting milk production. Management typically focuses on maintaining disease control while ensuring medication compatibility with breastfeeding. Many autoimmune therapies are compatible with lactation, though individualized evaluation is required. Fatigue associated with chronic illness may reduce feeding frequency if adequate support is not available, emphasizing the importance of social and clinical assistance. Newborn hypoglycemia, particularly in infants of diabetic mothers or those born small or large for gestational age, presents an immediate postpartum concern. Early initiation of breastfeeding promotes stabilization of blood glucose through provision of lactose and stimulation of endogenous regulatory mechanisms. Colostrum, though produced in small volumes, is concentrated and sufficient for most healthy term infants when feeds are frequent and effective. Monitoring protocols should prioritize maintaining maternal-infant proximity and supporting breastfeeding whenever possible rather than defaulting to separation. Supplementation decisions must balance metabolic safety with preservation of milk supply. Understanding the interaction between autoimmune physiology, endocrine balance, and neonatal glucose regulation enables targeted support that protects both maternal health and infant metabolic stability while sustaining effective lactation.

Download Audio file and flashcards

Chapter-3: Pathology

Ankyloglossia and Oral Restrictions

Ankyloglossia, commonly referred to as tongue-tie, is characterized by a restrictive lingual frenulum that limits tongue mobility and may interfere with effective breastfeeding. The tongue plays a central role in milk transfer by elevating, extending, and cupping around the nipple to create negative pressure and coordinated peristaltic motion. When tongue movement is restricted, the infant may be unable to achieve a deep latch, resulting in shallow attachment, nipple compression, and inadequate milk removal. Clinical signs often include maternal nipple pain, visible nipple distortion after feeding, clicking sounds during sucking, prolonged feeding sessions, poor weight gain, and infant frustration at the breast. Assessment must focus on functional impairment rather than appearance alone, as frenulum morphology varies widely. A comprehensive oral examination evaluates tongue elevation, lateralization, extension beyond the lower gum line, and ability to maintain suction. Posterior tongue restrictions may be more subtle but can still significantly impair feeding mechanics. Untreated restriction may contribute to low milk supply due to ineffective milk removal and can lead to early breastfeeding cessation. Management begins with optimization of positioning and latch to maximize available mobility. If functional limitation persists and is associated with feeding dysfunction, referral for further evaluation and possible frenotomy may be appropriate. Post-procedure support is essential to retrain sucking patterns and protect milk supply. Differentiating between true functional restriction and normal anatomical variation requires skilled assessment to prevent unnecessary intervention while ensuring timely treatment when indicated.

Cleft Lip, Cleft Palate, and Craniofacial Conditions

Cleft lip, cleft palate, and other craniofacial anomalies significantly affect breastfeeding due to altered oral structure and impaired ability to generate negative intraoral pressure. Effective breastfeeding depends on the infant's capacity to seal the oral cavity around the breast and compress the lactiferous sinuses rhythmically. A cleft lip may compromise the anterior seal, whereas a cleft palate disrupts separation between the oral and nasal cavities, making suction generation difficult or impossible. The degree of impairment varies according to the size and location of the defect. Infants with isolated cleft lip may breastfeed successfully with positioning adjustments that improve seal and stability. In contrast, those with cleft palate often require alternative feeding strategies because they cannot sustain adequate suction. Breast milk remains the optimal nutrition for these infants due to its immunologic and developmental benefits, and expressed milk can be provided using specialized feeding devices that compensate for reduced suction capacity. Feeding sessions may require pacing and upright positioning to reduce nasal regurgitation and aspiration risk. Close monitoring of weight gain and hydration status is essential. Surgical repair timing influences feeding management, and collaboration with multidisciplinary craniofacial teams ensures coordinated care. Emotional support for families is critical, as feeding challenges may be distressing. While direct breastfeeding may not always be feasible in cases of significant palatal involvement, maintaining maternal milk supply through consistent expression preserves the opportunity for breast contact and supports optimal nutritional outcomes.

Congenital and Gastrointestinal Anomalies

Congenital and gastrointestinal anomalies can significantly impact feeding tolerance and milk transfer. Structural conditions such as esophageal atresia, tracheoesophageal fistula, pyloric stenosis, and intestinal malrotation interfere with normal swallowing and digestion. Esophageal atresia prevents effective passage of milk from the oropharynx to the stomach, often necessitating surgical correction before oral feeding is established. Tracheoesophageal fistula increases aspiration risk, requiring careful airway protection and coordinated medical management. Pyloric stenosis presents with projectile vomiting due to gastric outlet obstruction and typically requires surgical intervention; until corrected, effective breastfeeding may be compromised due to inadequate gastric emptying. Gastrointestinal motility disorders can lead to feeding intolerance, abdominal distension, or reflux-like symptoms. In these contexts, expressed human milk is often preferred because of its digestibility and protective properties. Infants with congenital heart disease or other systemic anomalies may experience fatigue during feeds due to increased metabolic demands and reduced endurance. Shorter, more frequent feeding sessions or partial supplementation may be required while preserving maternal milk supply. Assessment must differentiate between normal feeding variation and pathology requiring medical intervention. Weight gain patterns, stool characteristics, emesis frequency, and feeding endurance provide critical diagnostic clues. Lactation management in the presence of congenital anomalies requires close collaboration with pediatric specialists to ensure safety while prioritizing continued access to human milk.

Gastroesophageal Reflux and GERD

Gastroesophageal reflux refers to the passage of gastric contents into the esophagus and is common in infancy due to immature lower esophageal sphincter tone. Physiologic reflux often peaks around two to four months of age and typically resolves as neuromuscular maturation improves. Infants may regurgitate small amounts of milk without discomfort and maintain appropriate weight gain. In contrast, gastroesophageal reflux disease involves symptomatic reflux associated with poor weight gain, feeding refusal, irritability, or respiratory complications. Distinguishing between physiologic reflux and disease is essential to prevent unnecessary medicalization. Breastfed infants may experience less severe reflux due to faster gastric emptying of human milk compared with artificial substitutes. Management of uncomplicated reflux includes maintaining upright positioning after feeds, avoiding overfeeding, and supporting effective latch to reduce air intake. Frequent, smaller feeds may improve tolerance in symptomatic infants. Excessive maternal dietary restriction is rarely indicated unless clear evidence of food protein intolerance exists. Pharmacologic treatment is reserved for severe cases and should be guided by pediatric evaluation. Overdiagnosis of reflux can undermine breastfeeding confidence and lead to premature supplementation. Thorough feeding assessment, growth monitoring, and parental education help differentiate normal developmental patterns from clinically significant disease while preserving breastfeeding whenever possible.

Hyperbilirubinemia and Jaundice Management

Hyperbilirubinemia in the newborn period arises from elevated serum bilirubin due to increased red blood cell turnover and immature hepatic conjugation pathways. Physiologic jaundice typically appears after 24 hours of age and peaks between days three and five in term infants. Adequate milk intake promotes bilirubin excretion through stooling; therefore, suboptimal feeding may exacerbate jaundice. Breastfeeding-associated jaundice can occur in the first week when milk transfer is insufficient, leading to decreased stool output and increased enterohepatic circulation of bilirubin. Early and frequent feeding reduces this risk by stimulating meconium passage and enhancing hydration. A separate entity, breast milk jaundice, appears later and is thought to involve factors in mature milk that influence bilirubin metabolism; it generally occurs in thriving infants and rarely requires interruption of breastfeeding. Clinical management focuses on monitoring bilirubin levels relative to age in hours and assessing feeding adequacy. Phototherapy is used when levels exceed treatment thresholds and can usually be implemented without discontinuing breastfeeding. Supplementation decisions must weigh the need for rapid bilirubin reduction against the importance of maintaining milk supply. Lactation support includes optimizing latch, increasing feeding frequency, and monitoring elimination patterns. Prompt identification and management prevent severe complications while reinforcing the role of effective breastfeeding in bilirubin clearance.

Neurological Disabilities and Feeding Implications

Neurological disabilities can significantly affect breastfeeding due to disruptions in muscle tone, coordination, reflex integration, and endurance. Effective feeding requires synchronized suck-swallow-breathe coordination regulated by central nervous system pathways. Conditions such as hypoxic-ischemic encephalopathy, cerebral palsy, intracranial hemorrhage, and genetic syndromes may impair oral motor control and compromise safe swallowing. Hypotonia may result in weak suction and poor latch stability, while hypertonia may cause jaw clenching or disorganized sucking patterns. Infants with neurologic impairment often fatigue quickly, leading to prolonged feeds with limited milk transfer. Inconsistent swallowing may increase risk of aspiration, particularly if protective airway reflexes are diminished. Assessment requires careful observation of feeding rhythm, respiratory stability, color changes, and signs of stress such as finger splaying or arching. Collaboration with speech and feeding specialists may be necessary to evaluate swallow safety. Human milk remains the optimal nutrition due to its immunologic properties and digestibility, especially for medically complex infants. Positioning adjustments, such as semi-upright or side-lying positions, may enhance airway protection and improve coordination. Some infants benefit from paced feeding techniques that allow breathing pauses. When direct breastfeeding is not immediately safe, expressed milk can be provided while oral skills are supported through non-nutritive sucking at the breast. Family counseling is critical, as neurologic diagnoses can create significant emotional distress. Early, individualized feeding plans that prioritize safety while maintaining maternal milk supply promote optimal developmental and nutritional outcomes.

Infant Infections and Vertically Transmitted Diseases

Infectious conditions in infancy may influence feeding tolerance, energy expenditure, and breastfeeding management. Many common neonatal infections, including viral respiratory illnesses, can temporarily reduce feeding endurance due to nasal congestion or increased metabolic demands. Breastfeeding provides immunologic protection through antibodies, leukocytes, and bioactive factors that support immune response and intestinal integrity. Continuation of breastfeeding during mild illness is generally recommended, as human milk enhances recovery and maintains hydration. In cases of vertically transmitted infections such as certain viral or bacterial diseases, management depends on pathogen type, maternal treatment status, and transmission risk through milk. Some infections require temporary precautions or specific therapeutic coordination, while others are compatible with continued breastfeeding. Careful evaluation of maternal medications ensures safety during treatment. Infants with systemic infection may demonstrate lethargy, poor suck, or decreased appetite, requiring close monitoring of intake and hydration. Hospitalized infants benefit from access to expressed milk if direct breastfeeding is not feasible. Education should emphasize that abrupt weaning during infection may reduce immune support and complicate recovery. Collaboration with pediatric infectious disease specialists ensures that feeding recommendations align with current evidence while preserving the benefits of human milk whenever safely possible.

Maternal Mastitis, Abscess, and Inflammatory Conditions

Mastitis is an inflammatory condition of the breast often associated with milk stasis and, in some cases, bacterial infection. It typically presents with localized breast pain, erythema, warmth, fever, and flu-like symptoms. Ineffective milk removal, infrequent feeding, abrupt weaning, or pressure from tight clothing may contribute to milk stasis, creating an environment conducive to inflammation. Early management focuses on improving milk drainage through frequent feeding or pumping, optimizing latch, and addressing any mechanical factors impairing milk removal. Continued breastfeeding from the affected breast is generally recommended, as milk removal aids resolution and does not pose risk to the healthy term infant in most cases. Supportive measures include rest, hydration, and anti-inflammatory therapy when indicated. If symptoms do not improve or worsen, antibiotic treatment targeting common pathogens may be required. Untreated mastitis can progress to abscess formation, characterized by localized fluctuance and persistent fever. Abscess management may involve drainage procedures while maintaining milk expression to preserve supply. Inflammatory breast conditions require prompt attention to prevent recurrence and protect lactation. Identifying underlying contributors such as nipple trauma, oversupply, or incomplete emptying reduces future risk. Comprehensive care integrates symptom management, milk supply preservation, and maternal well-being.

Milk Supply Disorders, Nipple Trauma, and Maternal Systemic Disease

Milk supply disorders encompass both insufficient and excessive production and often arise from a combination of physiologic, mechanical, and systemic factors. Primary insufficient glandular tissue may limit maximal production capacity, whereas secondary low supply more commonly results from ineffective milk removal, delayed lactogenesis, endocrine imbalance, or supplementation without adequate stimulation. Signs of low supply include poor infant weight gain, decreased elimination, and minimal breast fullness. Evaluation requires assessment of latch quality, feeding frequency, maternal endocrine history, and infant oral function. Management centers on increasing effective milk removal through frequent feeding or pumping and addressing underlying causes. Hyperlactation, or oversupply, may present with breast engorgement, forceful let-down, infant choking, and green frothy stools due to foremilk-hindmilk imbalance during rapid flow. Controlled milk removal strategies may help regulate production. Nipple trauma commonly results from shallow latch or improper positioning and may manifest as cracks, bleeding, or persistent pain. Correction of latch mechanics is essential for healing and prevention of infection. Maternal systemic diseases such as anemia, thyroid dysfunction, or autoimmune conditions may indirectly influence milk production through metabolic or hormonal pathways. Comprehensive assessment distinguishes between local mechanical issues and systemic contributors. Protecting milk supply while addressing maternal health conditions ensures sustainable breastfeeding and prevents premature cessation.

Chapter-4 : Pharmacology and Toxicology

Alcohol and Lactation

Alcohol consumption during lactation raises important pharmacokinetic and clinical considerations. Ethanol is a small, water-soluble molecule that passes readily from maternal plasma into human milk by passive diffusion. Milk alcohol concentration closely parallels maternal blood alcohol concentration, meaning that levels rise and fall in tandem rather than accumulating in milk. Alcohol is not stored in breast tissue; therefore, strategies such as discarding expressed milk do not accelerate elimination from the body. Metabolism occurs primarily in the liver at a relatively constant rate, influenced by body weight, hepatic function, and amount consumed. Peak levels typically occur within 30 to 60 minutes after ingestion on an empty stomach and may be delayed if consumed with food. From a physiologic perspective, alcohol may transiently inhibit oxytocin release, potentially reducing milk ejection and temporarily decreasing infant milk intake during feeding sessions occurring at peak levels. Some infants may demonstrate altered sleep patterns or decreased feeding vigor following exposure. Chronic or heavy alcohol use may impair milk production and affect infant neurodevelopment, particularly with repeated high exposure. Occasional moderate consumption can be managed by timing feeds to minimize infant exposure, allowing sufficient time for maternal metabolism before the next feeding. Education should emphasize that maternal impairment affects caregiving safety independently of milk transfer considerations. Counseling must balance risk awareness with avoidance of unnecessary breastfeeding interruption, as abrupt cessation may compromise milk supply. Individualized guidance supports informed decision-making while preserving lactation whenever safely possible.

Nicotine, Tobacco, and Vaping

Nicotine exposure during lactation occurs primarily through tobacco smoking, smokeless tobacco products, and electronic nicotine delivery systems. Nicotine is rapidly absorbed into maternal circulation and transfers into human milk, where concentrations may exceed maternal plasma levels due to ion trapping in the slightly acidic milk environment. The half-life of nicotine in milk is relatively short, yet repeated exposure through frequent smoking leads to sustained infant exposure. Nicotine may alter infant sleep patterns, increase irritability, and affect cardiovascular regulation. Smoking is also associated with reduced milk production, possibly through dopaminergic inhibition of prolactin secretion. Additionally, tobacco smoke exposure increases risk of sudden infant death syndrome, respiratory infections, and asthma. Despite these risks, breastfeeding remains beneficial compared with formula feeding in smoking individuals, as human milk provides immunologic protection that may mitigate some respiratory complications. Counseling focuses on harm reduction, including smoking cessation support, minimizing exposure through smoking immediately after rather than before feeding, avoiding indoor smoking, and changing clothing before infant contact to reduce third-hand smoke exposure. Electronic nicotine delivery systems introduce additional concerns related to variable nicotine concentrations and potential exposure to flavoring chemicals. Long-term safety data are limited. The priority remains cessation of nicotine use; however, when cessation is not immediately achievable, continuation of breastfeeding with exposure mitigation strategies generally provides greater overall benefit than discontinuation of lactation.

Cannabis and Breastfeeding

Cannabis contains psychoactive compounds, including delta-9-tetrahydrocannabinol (THC), which are highly lipophilic and readily accumulate in fatty tissues, including breast milk. Due to its lipid solubility, THC may persist in milk for extended periods compared with substances such as alcohol. Transfer into milk occurs through passive diffusion, and repeated use can result in accumulation, leading to ongoing infant exposure even when maternal plasma levels decline. The developing infant brain is particularly sensitive to neuroactive compounds, and theoretical concerns include potential effects on neurodevelopment, motor function, and executive functioning. Evidence regarding long-term outcomes remains limited and sometimes confounded by prenatal exposure and environmental variables. Cannabis use may also alter maternal responsiveness and caregiving capacity if cognitive or psychomotor impairment occurs. Additionally, smoking cannabis exposes infants to combustion byproducts similar to tobacco smoke. Counseling requires a nonjudgmental approach that provides clear information regarding potential risks while encouraging cessation or reduction. If use continues, strategies to minimize exposure include avoiding direct smoke contact and refraining from breastfeeding during periods of acute intoxication. Because of prolonged persistence in milk, timing feeds may not fully eliminate exposure risk. Lactation professionals must remain aware of evolving research and legal contexts while prioritizing infant safety and maternal support.

Drugs of Abuse and Substance Use Disorders

Substance use disorders involving opioids, stimulants, sedatives, and other illicit drugs present complex challenges in lactation management. Many substances cross into human milk to varying degrees depending on molecular weight, lipid solubility, protein binding, and half-life. Opioids such as heroin and non-prescribed synthetic opioids can cause infant sedation, respiratory depression, and poor feeding if transferred in significant amounts. Stimulants such as cocaine and methamphetamine may lead to irritability, tachycardia, and neurotoxicity. The unpredictable purity and potency of illicit substances increase risk of adverse effects. In contrast, medication-assisted treatment for opioid use disorder, when appropriately prescribed and monitored, is often compatible with breastfeeding and may reduce severity of neonatal abstinence symptoms. Stable participation in treatment programs, absence of ongoing illicit use, and consistent prenatal care influence recommendations. Breastfeeding provides benefits including enhanced maternal-infant bonding and improved neurobehavioral outcomes in some contexts. However, active uncontrolled substance use with ongoing intoxication generally contraindicates direct breastfeeding due to safety concerns. Multidisciplinary collaboration involving addiction specialists, pediatric providers, and lactation professionals ensures individualized care plans. Compassionate, stigma-free counseling encourages disclosure and engagement in treatment, which ultimately supports safer parenting and feeding practices.

Prescription and Over-the-Counter Medications

Most prescription and over-the-counter medications are compatible with breastfeeding, but evaluation requires understanding pharmacokinetic principles. Transfer into milk depends on molecular size, lipid solubility, ionization, protein binding, and half-life. Medications with high protein binding and large molecular weight typically transfer in minimal amounts. The relative infant dose, calculated as the infant's dose through milk divided by the maternal weight-adjusted dose, provides a standardized measure of exposure. In general, relative infant doses below 10 percent are considered acceptable for most medications, though clinical context is essential. Timing of doses relative to feeding may reduce infant exposure for drugs with short half-lives. Particular caution is warranted with medications that cause central nervous system depression, prolonged half-life, or active metabolites. Premature or medically fragile infants may have reduced drug clearance and require additional consideration. Abrupt discontinuation of necessary maternal medication may pose greater risk than continued breastfeeding with monitored exposure. Individualized risk-benefit analysis guides decision-making. Access to up-to-date pharmacologic resources supports evidence-based counseling. Clear communication with prescribing providers ensures coordinated care that protects both maternal health and infant safety while maintaining lactation whenever possible.

Labor and Delivery Medications

Medications administered during labor and delivery may influence early breastfeeding through effects on neonatal alertness, maternal responsiveness, and hormonal transitions. Analgesics, anesthetics, and synthetic oxytocin are commonly used in intrapartum care, and each has distinct pharmacologic properties that affect the immediate postpartum period. Opioid analgesics cross the placenta and may result in transient neonatal respiratory depression, decreased alertness, and impaired suck reflex during the first hours after birth. Epidural anesthesia typically results in lower systemic exposure than intravenous opioids, but higher cumulative doses may still contribute to delayed initiation of effective feeding in some dyads. General anesthesia used during cesarean birth may prolong neonatal sleepiness, although most healthy term infants can breastfeed once alert and stable. Synthetic oxytocin administered for induction or augmentation of labor may alter endogenous oxytocin receptor dynamics, though clinical implications for lactation vary. Early skin-to-skin contact and uninterrupted access to the breast mitigate many medication-related effects by stimulating physiologic hormonal responses and promoting neonatal reflexes. When infants demonstrate decreased alertness, strategies such as hand expression, gentle stimulation, and frequent feeding attempts support lactation establishment. Monitoring for delayed lactogenesis II is appropriate in cases involving prolonged labor, significant blood loss, or extensive pharmacologic exposure. Education should reassure families that most intrapartum medications are compatible with breastfeeding and that early challenges are often temporary. Proactive support during the first 24 to 48 hours enhances successful transition to effective feeding despite medication exposure.

Contraception and Hormonal Influence

Postpartum contraception must be selected with consideration of its potential impact on milk production and infant exposure. Estrogen-containing contraceptives may reduce milk supply, particularly when initiated before lactation is well established, due to estrogen's inhibitory effect on prolactin-mediated milk synthesis. For this reason, combined hormonal contraceptives are generally delayed until lactation is stable and infant growth is well established. Progestin-only methods, including pills, injectables, and implants, are often preferred during early lactation because they have minimal effect on milk production when initiated after the immediate postpartum period. Intrauterine devices, both hormonal and non-hormonal, provide effective long-term contraception with negligible systemic hormone levels in the case of non-hormonal devices and minimal transfer into milk with progestin-releasing systems. Lactational amenorrhea itself provides temporary contraceptive protection when strict criteria are met, including exclusive breastfeeding, amenorrhea, and infant age under six months; however, efficacy declines once supplemental feeding begins or menses resume. Counseling should emphasize that individual responses to hormonal contraception vary, and monitoring milk supply after initiation is prudent. If decreased supply is suspected, alternative methods may be considered. Balancing contraceptive efficacy with preservation of lactation requires individualized assessment and informed decision-making that supports both reproductive planning and breastfeeding continuation.

Galactagogues and Milk Supply Agents

Galactagogues are substances used to stimulate milk production and may include pharmaceutical agents, herbal preparations, and nutritional supplements. Pharmacologic galactagogues often function by increasing prolactin levels through dopamine antagonism, thereby enhancing stimulation of mammary receptors. However, elevated prolactin alone does not guarantee sustained milk production if effective milk removal is inadequate. Therefore, optimization of feeding frequency and latch mechanics remains the cornerstone of supply management before pharmacologic intervention is considered. Herbal galactagogues such as fenugreek and other botanicals are widely used, though evidence regarding efficacy and safety varies in quality and consistency. Some individuals report subjective increases in milk volume, while others experience no effect or adverse reactions. Potential side effects may include gastrointestinal discomfort or allergic responses. Dosage standardization is often lacking in herbal products, making consistent evaluation challenging. Before recommending any galactagogue, clinicians must assess underlying causes of low supply, including endocrine disorders, retained placental fragments, insufficient glandular tissue, or ineffective milk transfer. Use of galactagogues without addressing primary causes may delay appropriate intervention. In some cases, short-term pharmacologic support may assist in establishing supply while mechanical stimulation continues. Counseling should present realistic expectations, emphasizing that galactagogues are adjunctive rather than primary therapies. Continuous monitoring of infant weight gain and maternal response guides ongoing management decisions.

Herbs, Supplements, and Alternative Therapies

Herbal products and dietary supplements are frequently used during lactation for a variety of indications, including perceived milk enhancement, mood support, and general wellness. Unlike prescription medications, many supplements are not subject to rigorous regulatory oversight, leading to variability in purity, concentration, and contamination risk. Transfer into human milk depends on molecular characteristics similar to those governing pharmaceutical agents, but robust pharmacokinetic data are often limited. Some herbal preparations may contain active compounds capable of affecting infant physiology, including sedation or gastrointestinal disturbance. Additionally, interactions between supplements and prescription medications may alter efficacy or safety. Alternative therapies such as homeopathy, acupuncture, or dietary regimens may be pursued by some families; while certain modalities pose minimal direct risk, they should not replace evidence-based management of medical conditions affecting lactation. Clinicians must inquire routinely about supplement use to identify potential exposures. Counseling should focus on evidence appraisal, encouraging use of reputable products when chosen and avoiding substances with known toxicity or insufficient safety data. Emphasizing that "natural" does not automatically equate to safe is important in preventing inadvertent harm. A balanced approach supports informed choice while prioritizing maternal and infant safety.

Chemotherapy, Radiation, and Diagnostic Exposures

Cancer treatment and diagnostic imaging introduce complex considerations for lactation. Many chemotherapeutic agents are cytotoxic and can transfer into human milk at levels potentially harmful to the infant. Due to their mechanisms of action targeting rapidly dividing cells, exposure through milk may pose significant risk, and breastfeeding is generally contraindicated during active chemotherapy. Temporary cessation with maintenance of milk expression may be considered in certain circumstances depending on drug half-life and treatment schedule, but careful coordination with oncology specialists is essential. Radiation therapy directed away from the breast typically does not contaminate milk; however, radiation involving breast tissue may reduce milk production in the treated breast due to glandular damage. Diagnostic imaging procedures using non-radioactive contrast agents are often compatible with continued breastfeeding, as transfer into milk is minimal and oral bioavailability in the infant is low. Radioactive isotopes used in certain scans may require temporary interruption of breastfeeding until radioactivity decays to safe levels. Clear, individualized guidance prevents unnecessary long-term cessation when only brief interruption is required. Emotional support is critical, as concurrent cancer diagnosis and lactation concerns can be profoundly distressing. Protecting infant safety while supporting maternal treatment and, when possible, preserving future lactation potential requires coordinated interdisciplinary care.

Chapter-5: Psychology, Sociology, and Anthropology

Transition to Parenthood and Identity Development

The transition to parenthood represents a profound biopsychosocial transformation that influences breastfeeding initiation, continuation, and overall family adjustment. This developmental period involves shifts in identity, roles, relationships, and daily routines. Individuals must integrate the parental role into their existing sense of self while adapting to physical recovery, sleep disruption, and increased caregiving responsibility. Breastfeeding often becomes central to this identity formation, serving as both a nurturing act and a visible marker of parenting competence. Positive early feeding experiences may reinforce confidence and attachment, whereas difficulties can trigger self-doubt and emotional distress. Societal expectations regarding ideal parenting practices may intensify pressure, particularly when individuals perceive breastfeeding as a measure of success. Hormonal fluctuations in the postpartum period also influence mood, emotional sensitivity, and stress regulation, interacting with psychosocial factors. Supportive environments that validate effort rather than outcome foster resilience and adaptive coping. Partners and family members play critical roles in shaping maternal confidence through practical assistance and emotional affirmation. Cultural narratives about motherhood influence expectations surrounding self-sacrifice, productivity, and feeding norms. When the transition is complicated by medical issues, traumatic birth experiences, or lack of support, the risk of early breastfeeding cessation increases. Lactation professionals must assess not only technical feeding mechanics but also the psychological adjustment process. Providing anticipatory guidance regarding common emotional fluctuations normalizes experience and reduces isolation. Empowerment-based counseling that recognizes parental strengths promotes self-efficacy. Understanding the transition to parenthood as a developmental process rather than a single event enables more comprehensive support that protects both emotional well-being and breastfeeding continuity.

Maternal Mental Health and Mood Disorders

Maternal mental health significantly influences breastfeeding outcomes, and mood disorders in the perinatal period require careful identification and management. Postpartum blues, characterized by transient mood lability and tearfulness in the first week after birth, are common and typically self-limited. In contrast, postpartum depression involves persistent sadness, loss of interest, sleep disturbance beyond expected newborn-related disruption, and potential feelings of inadequacy or hopelessness. Anxiety disorders may manifest as excessive worry about infant health, intrusive thoughts, or physiological hyperarousal. These conditions can interfere with feeding confidence, milk ejection reflex responsiveness, and consistency of feeding routines. Hormonal changes, prior psychiatric history, traumatic birth experiences, and inadequate social support contribute to risk. Breastfeeding itself may exert protective effects for some individuals through oxytocin-mediated stress reduction and enhanced bonding; however, when feeding difficulties coexist with depression or anxiety, stress may intensify symptoms. Screening tools administered during postpartum visits support early detection. Treatment may include psychotherapy, social support interventions, and when indicated, pharmacologic therapy compatible with lactation. Abrupt discontinuation of breastfeeding solely due to maternal medication use is rarely necessary when appropriate agents are selected. Stigma surrounding mental health may deter disclosure, making nonjudgmental inquiry essential. Lactation professionals should remain vigilant for signs of mood disturbance, including flat affect, disengagement, or overwhelming guilt related to feeding. Timely referral to mental health providers ensures comprehensive care. Supporting maternal mental health not only enhances overall well-being but also strengthens the breastfeeding relationship and promotes healthy infant development.

Cognitive and Psychological Conditions

Cognitive and psychological conditions, including attention-deficit disorders, learning disabilities, trauma histories, and severe mental illness, may influence breastfeeding experiences through effects on executive functioning, emotional regulation, and daily organization. Individuals with attention or memory challenges may struggle with maintaining consistent feeding or pumping schedules, particularly in the context of sleep deprivation. Clear, structured care plans and written instructions can enhance adherence and reduce overwhelm. Trauma histories, including prior abuse or obstetric trauma, may be triggered by physical sensations associated with breastfeeding, leading to discomfort or dissociation during feeds. Sensitive, trauma-informed care prioritizes consent, control, and pacing to minimize retraumatization. Severe psychiatric conditions such as bipolar disorder or psychotic disorders require coordinated management to balance medication safety with maternal stability. Cognitive impairments may also affect comprehension of feeding cues or safe sleep guidance, necessitating tailored education strategies. Assessment should consider literacy level, cultural context, and preferred learning style. Breastfeeding may provide grounding and bonding benefits for some individuals with psychological vulnerabilities, yet rigid expectations may exacerbate stress. Flexibility in feeding plans that accommodates individual capacity supports sustained engagement. Collaboration with mental health professionals enhances continuity of care. Recognizing the diverse cognitive and psychological profiles among parents allows individualized support that preserves both safety and dignity while promoting successful lactation where desired.

Breastfeeding Dyad Attachment and Bonding

Breastfeeding contributes to attachment formation through repeated cycles of proximity, eye contact, tactile stimulation, and hormonal reinforcement. Oxytocin release during feeding enhances maternal relaxation and affiliative behaviors while supporting infant emotional regulation. Secure attachment develops through consistent responsiveness to infant cues, not solely through feeding method; however, breastfeeding provides frequent opportunities for synchronous interaction. Early skin-to-skin contact promotes physiologic stabilization and initiates bonding pathways immediately after birth. Sensitive interpretation of hunger cues and prompt feeding reinforce infant trust and caregiver competence. Challenges such as latch difficulties, pain, or medical complications may disrupt these interactions and generate frustration within the dyad. Interventions that restore comfort and feeding effectiveness often improve relational harmony. Cultural expectations regarding independence, co-sleeping, and feeding frequency influence attachment practices and should be respected within safety guidelines. In cases of postpartum depression or maternal stress, bonding may be impaired; breastfeeding support that reduces discomfort and enhances confidence can indirectly strengthen attachment. Conversely, when breastfeeding becomes a source of persistent distress, individualized counseling ensures that attachment goals are met regardless of feeding modality. The quality of relational interaction rather than exclusive feeding status ultimately shapes secure attachment. Lactation professionals must consider the dyad as an integrated system, recognizing that feeding support extends beyond nutrition to encompass emotional connection and developmental security.

Cultural Beliefs and Feeding Practices

Cultural beliefs profoundly shape perceptions of breastfeeding, acceptable duration, supplementation practices, and maternal roles. In some cultures, colostrum is highly valued for its protective qualities, while in others it may be discarded due to misconceptions about purity. Rituals surrounding birth and postpartum confinement may influence early feeding frequency and maternal rest. Extended family members often hold influential roles in guiding feeding decisions, and intergenerational advice may conflict with contemporary recommendations. Cultural norms regarding modesty affect comfort with public breastfeeding and may influence feeding patterns outside the home. Work expectations, community infrastructure, and social attitudes toward breastfeeding in public spaces further shape practice. Migration and acculturation can create tension between traditional feeding practices and host-country norms. Lactation support must be culturally responsive, acknowledging values without imposing judgment. Open-ended inquiry about family beliefs encourages collaborative care planning. Education should be framed within culturally meaningful contexts, emphasizing shared goals of infant health and family well-being. Failure to recognize cultural influences may result in miscommunication and decreased adherence to guidance. Respectful integration of cultural practices with evidence-based recommendations strengthens trust and improves breastfeeding outcomes across diverse populations.

Family Systems and Support Networks

Breastfeeding occurs within the context of family systems that shape parental confidence, decision-making, and sustainability of feeding practices. Family systems theory emphasizes that individuals do not function in isolation but within interconnected relational networks that influence behavior and coping. Partners, grandparents, extended relatives, and close friends may provide instrumental support such as meal preparation, infant care assistance, and household management, all of which indirectly protect milk supply by reducing maternal stress and fatigue. Emotional support, including encouragement and reassurance during feeding challenges, strengthens parental self-efficacy. Conversely, conflicting advice, skepticism about milk adequacy, or pressure to supplement may undermine confidence and disrupt exclusive breastfeeding. Intergenerational differences in infant feeding norms often reflect historical shifts in formula marketing, workplace patterns, and public health messaging. Addressing these dynamics requires respectful communication that validates family involvement while reinforcing evidence-based guidance. Inclusion of partners in lactation education enhances understanding of feeding cues, normal newborn behavior, and ways to participate in caregiving beyond feeding. Social isolation, particularly in nuclear family settings or among recent migrants, may limit access to experienced role models, increasing vulnerability to early cessation. Peer support groups and community-based networks provide normalization and shared problem-solving opportunities. Assessing the quality and availability of support systems enables tailored interventions that strengthen protective factors. Breastfeeding success is strongly correlated with perceived support; therefore, fostering collaborative family engagement is a central component of effective lactation care.

Employment, Workplace Policy, and Lactation

Return to employment introduces structural and logistical challenges that significantly influence breastfeeding duration. Workplace culture, availability of private pumping spaces, schedule flexibility, and employer attitudes determine whether lactation can be maintained effectively. Milk production relies on regular removal; therefore, extended separation without opportunities for expression may reduce supply. Planning for return to work should begin during the prenatal or early postpartum period, including establishing a pumping routine, building a stored milk supply when desired, and discussing accommodations with employers. Legal protections in many regions mandate reasonable break time and private space for milk expression, though implementation varies. Shift work, physically demanding labor, and unpredictable schedules may complicate consistent pumping. Education regarding milk storage guidelines, pump maintenance, and time management enhances confidence. Emotional factors also influence continuation, as individuals may experience guilt, stress, or ambivalence balancing employment and caregiving roles. Supportive supervisors and colleagues positively affect lactation persistence. Telework arrangements or onsite childcare facilitate continued direct breastfeeding when feasible. Without institutional support, individuals may prematurely wean despite strong initial intentions. Advocacy for family-friendly workplace policies contributes to broader public health improvement. Addressing employment-related barriers proactively protects milk supply and supports sustained breastfeeding within the realities of modern work environments.

Birth Practices and Early Feeding Influence

Birth practices exert a significant influence on early breastfeeding outcomes through their effects on maternal physiology, neonatal alertness, and immediate postpartum contact. Immediate and uninterrupted skin-to-skin contact promotes thermoregulation, stabilizes neonatal glucose levels, and stimulates instinctive feeding behaviors. Delayed cord clamping supports neonatal iron stores and circulatory adaptation, indirectly contributing to feeding readiness. Conversely, routine separation, excessive suctioning, or unnecessary procedures may disrupt the infant's innate progression toward self-attachment. Mode of birth also plays a role; cesarean delivery may delay maternal mobility and increase discomfort, potentially affecting early positioning and frequency of feeding. However, with adequate support, successful breastfeeding is achievable following both vaginal and surgical births. Use of intrapartum medications may temporarily influence neonatal alertness, necessitating additional stimulation and patience during initial feeds. Rooming-in policies facilitate cue-based feeding and reduce reliance on supplementation. Early formula supplementation without medical indication may interfere with milk supply establishment by reducing breast stimulation. Education of healthcare staff and families regarding physiologic newborn behavior reduces misinterpretation of normal cluster feeding or sleep patterns. Birth environment policies that prioritize maternal-infant proximity and minimize unnecessary intervention enhance early feeding success. Understanding the interplay between obstetric care and lactation physiology enables advocacy for practices that support optimal breastfeeding initiation.

Safe Sleep and Infant Care Practices

Safe sleep recommendations intersect with breastfeeding practices and influence nighttime feeding patterns. Placing infants on their backs on a firm, separate sleep surface reduces risk of sleep-related infant deaths. Room-sharing without bed-sharing is commonly recommended to facilitate responsive nighttime feeding while maintaining safety. Breastfeeding itself is associated with reduced risk of sudden infant death, potentially due to immunologic protection and more arousable sleep states. Night feeding supports prolactin secretion and helps maintain milk supply, particularly in early infancy. Parental fatigue, however, may increase risk of unsafe sleep arrangements if not proactively addressed. Education regarding safe positioning, avoidance of soft bedding, and recognition of infant sleep cues promotes protective behaviors. Cultural norms surrounding co-sleeping vary, and counseling must balance safety guidance with respectful dialogue. Pacifier use during sleep has been associated with reduced sudden infant death risk, though introduction timing may influence breastfeeding establishment. Clear, evidence-based counseling empowers families to make informed decisions that protect both infant safety and lactation continuity. Integrating safe sleep education into lactation support ensures consistent messaging and reinforces that breastfeeding and safe sleep practices are complementary components of infant care.

Weaning Across Developmental Stages

Weaning is a developmental process rather than a single event and may occur gradually or abruptly depending on family preference, infant readiness, and contextual factors. Natural or child-led weaning often unfolds over months as solid food intake increases and nursing frequency decreases. Developmental milestones such as increased mobility, language acquisition, and social engagement may shift the function of breastfeeding from primary nutrition to comfort and connection. Abrupt weaning may be initiated due to maternal illness, return to work, pregnancy, or personal choice and can carry emotional and physiologic implications. Rapid cessation may lead to breast engorgement, mastitis risk, and emotional distress for both parent and child. Gradual reduction of feeds allows physiologic downregulation of milk production through autocrine mechanisms. Emotional responses to weaning vary widely and may include relief, sadness, or ambivalence. Cultural norms strongly influence acceptable duration of breastfeeding and perceptions of extended nursing. Supportive counseling normalizes diverse experiences and emphasizes that healthy attachment does not depend on a specific weaning age. When weaning is medically necessary, guidance on milk expression tapering and comfort measures protects maternal health. Understanding weaning as a relational and biologic transition enables compassionate support tailored to individual family goals and circumstances.

Chapter-6: Techniques

The First Hour and Early Initiation

The first hour after birth represents a critical window for breastfeeding initiation, often referred to as the sensitive period for neonatal adaptation and maternal-infant bonding. During this time, healthy term infants placed skin-to-skin with the birthing parent demonstrate a predictable sequence of instinctive behaviors including alertness, hand-to-mouth movements, rooting, crawling toward the breast, and self-attachment. These behaviors are biologically programmed and facilitated by uninterrupted contact. Early initiation stimulates oxytocin release, promoting uterine contraction, reducing postpartum bleeding, and enhancing milk ejection reflex responsiveness. It also stimulates prolactin receptor activity in the mammary gland, supporting long-term milk production. Delays in first feeding due to separation, routine procedures, or medical interventions may interfere with this natural progression and increase risk of supplementation. Even when medical complications occur, early hand expression of colostrum within the first hour can initiate lactation physiology and provide immunologically rich milk for the infant. For infants who are sleepy or affected by labor medications, gentle stimulation and patience support feeding readiness without forceful attempts. Observing feeding cues rather than imposing rigid schedules respects newborn neurobehavioral patterns. The first feeding session may vary in duration and effectiveness; the goal is not perfection but stimulation and exposure. Early skin-to-skin contact enhances thermoregulation, glucose stability, and respiratory adaptation, all of which support feeding capacity. Establishing breastfeeding during this period sets the foundation for supply regulation and maternal confidence. Proactive support in the immediate postpartum environment is therefore a cornerstone of successful lactation establishment.

Skin-to-Skin (Kangaroo Care)

Skin-to-skin contact, often referred to as kangaroo care, involves placing the unclothed infant prone on the caregiver's bare chest, promoting physiologic stability and breastfeeding success. This practice supports thermoregulation through conductive heat transfer, stabilizes heart rate and respiratory patterns, and enhances neonatal glucose regulation. Skin-to-skin contact stimulates oxytocin release, which strengthens bonding and supports milk ejection. In the early postpartum period, continuous contact facilitates recognition of feeding cues and increases frequency of spontaneous latching attempts. For preterm infants, kangaroo care has been associated with improved weight gain, enhanced cardiorespiratory stability, and earlier transition to direct breastfeeding. The sensory environment created by skin-to-skin positioning, including maternal scent and heartbeat, promotes neurodevelopmental organization and reduces stress responses. Skin-to-skin contact is beneficial beyond the immediate postpartum period and can be used to calm infants, encourage feeding after periods of separation, and support relactation efforts. It also assists in regulating infant state transitions, increasing quiet alert periods during which feeding is most effective. Barriers to implementation may include institutional routines or parental discomfort; education regarding safety and benefits improves acceptance. Safe positioning requires that the infant's airway remains clear, with head turned to the side and neck slightly extended. Encouraging regular skin-to-skin sessions strengthens lactation physiology and enhances the relational aspects of breastfeeding.

Positioning and Hands-Off Techniques

Effective positioning facilitates deep latch, efficient milk transfer, and maternal comfort. Optimal positioning aligns the infant's ear, shoulder, and hip in a straight line, with the body turned toward the breast to prevent neck rotation. The infant's nose should align with the nipple before latch, encouraging a wide gape and asymmetric attachment that includes more areolar tissue below the nipple than above. Common positions include cradle, cross-cradle, football hold, and side-lying, each offering specific advantages depending on maternal anatomy, infant size, and medical circumstances. Hands-off techniques emphasize supporting the dyad in achieving effective positioning without excessive manual manipulation of the breast or infant's head. Encouraging the infant to self-attach when possible respects innate feeding reflexes and may reduce nipple trauma associated with forced latch. Maternal comfort is equally important; unsupported posture can lead to musculoskeletal strain and contribute to early discontinuation. Pillows or rolled blankets may provide stability while maintaining flexibility for infant movement. In cases of nipple pain or shallow latch, minor adjustments in angle or body alignment often resolve symptoms without invasive intervention. For individuals with larger breasts or post-surgical anatomy, additional support may be required to ensure adequate airway visibility and infant access. Mastery of positioning principles allows adaptation to diverse clinical scenarios and promotes sustainable, pain-free breastfeeding.

Latch Mechanics and Assessment

Latch quality directly influences milk transfer efficiency and maternal nipple integrity. A deep, asymmetric latch positions the nipple toward the junction of the hard and soft palate, allowing the tongue to extend over the lower gum ridge and create rhythmic peristaltic motion. Effective latch is characterized by wide mouth opening, flanged lips, rounded cheeks without dimpling, and audible swallowing after milk ejection. Pain beyond initial latch-on discomfort may indicate shallow attachment, tongue restriction, or misalignment. Visual assessment should include observation of jaw excursion, ear movement indicating active sucking, and sustained rhythmic pattern of suck-swallow-breathe coordination. Nipple shape after feeding provides additional information; a compressed or creased nipple suggests suboptimal positioning. Assessment must integrate maternal comfort, infant behavior, and objective indicators of milk transfer such as weight gain and elimination patterns. Correcting latch often involves repositioning the infant to achieve a wider gape, supporting the breast to facilitate deeper attachment, and waiting for spontaneous mouth opening before bringing the infant to the breast. Overly forceful attempts to achieve latch may increase resistance and stress. Skilled latch assessment prevents secondary complications including nipple trauma, mastitis, and low milk supply due to ineffective removal. Comprehensive evaluation ensures that mechanical factors are addressed promptly, preserving both comfort and lactation sustainability.

Effective Milk Transfer Evaluation

Evaluating milk transfer involves assessing both the mechanical process of feeding and the clinical outcomes that indicate adequate intake. Direct observation of feeding provides immediate information about latch depth, sucking rhythm, and swallowing frequency. Audible or visible swallowing after let-down suggests effective transfer, particularly when accompanied by steady jaw movement and relaxation of the infant's hands and body. Breast softening after feeding indicates milk removal, though perception of fullness varies among individuals. Pre- and post-feed weights using sensitive scales may quantify intake when concerns arise regarding weight gain or milk supply. However, such measurements should be interpreted within the broader clinical context rather than in isolation. Infant output patterns, including appropriate stooling and voiding frequency, provide indirect evidence of transfer. Behavioral cues such as contentment after feeding and appropriate wakefulness between feeds also inform assessment. Poor transfer may present as prolonged feeding sessions without swallowing, persistent fussiness, or inadequate weight gain. Contributing factors include shallow latch, oral anatomical restrictions, low milk supply, or ineffective sucking patterns. Management strategies depend on underlying cause and may include latch optimization, breast compressions to enhance flow, or supplemental feeding methods that preserve breastfeeding stimulation. Ongoing monitoring ensures that interventions effectively improve transfer and support healthy growth. Skilled evaluation of milk transfer is central to resolving feeding concerns and maintaining breastfeeding success.

Managing Low Milk Supply

Management of low milk supply requires systematic assessment to distinguish perceived insufficiency from true physiologic inadequate production. Perceived low supply is common and often arises from misunderstanding normal newborn behavior such as cluster feeding, frequent night waking, or shorter feeding sessions as infants become more efficient. True low supply may present with inadequate infant weight gain, decreased urine and stool output, persistent hunger cues after feeds, and minimal breast fullness changes. Evaluation begins with direct observation of feeding to assess latch depth, suck-swallow coordination, and milk transfer effectiveness. Ineffective milk removal is the most common cause of secondary low supply and must be addressed through positioning adjustments, increased feeding frequency, and, when necessary, supplemental pumping after feeds to enhance stimulation. Endocrine factors such as thyroid dysfunction, retained placental fragments, insulin resistance, or prior breast surgery should be considered when supply does not improve with optimized technique. Increasing feeding frequency to at least eight to twelve times per 24 hours enhances prolactin receptor activity and supports upregulation of milk synthesis. Breast compressions during feeding may improve flow and maintain infant engagement. When supplementation is medically necessary, methods that preserve breast stimulation are preferred to prevent further reduction in supply. Parental counseling should emphasize realistic expectations, as milk production responds gradually to increased demand. Emotional reassurance is critical, as anxiety can interfere with milk ejection and feeding consistency. A structured, evidence-based plan that addresses mechanical, hormonal, and behavioral components provides the greatest likelihood of restoring adequate milk production.

Managing Oversupply and Engorgement

Oversupply and engorgement represent conditions in which milk production exceeds infant demand or milk removal is temporarily impaired, leading to breast fullness, discomfort, and potential feeding difficulties. Engorgement commonly occurs in the early postpartum period as lactogenesis II progresses and vascular congestion contributes to breast firmness and edema. Severe engorgement may flatten the nipple, making latch more difficult and reducing effective milk transfer. Gentle, frequent feeding remains the primary intervention, as milk removal reduces intramammary pressure and restores comfort. Hand expression prior to latch may soften the areola, facilitating deeper attachment. Application of warmth before feeding and cool compresses afterward may relieve discomfort, while anti-inflammatory measures support symptom control. Chronic oversupply may manifest as forceful milk ejection, infant choking or coughing during feeds, excessive weight gain, and frothy green stools related to rapid transit of lactose-rich milk. In such cases, regulated milk removal strategies may be employed to gradually decrease production without abrupt suppression. Avoiding excessive pumping beyond infant needs prevents further stimulation that perpetuates oversupply. Management requires careful balance to prevent blocked ducts or mastitis resulting from incomplete emptying. Education regarding normal fullness versus pathologic engorgement reduces unnecessary intervention. A measured approach that aligns production with infant demand preserves maternal comfort while maintaining effective breastfeeding.

Medically Indicated Supplementation

Supplementation may be medically indicated in circumstances such as significant weight loss beyond expected physiologic norms, persistent hypoglycemia, dehydration, or delayed lactogenesis with inadequate intake. The decision to supplement should follow thorough assessment of feeding technique and milk transfer to ensure that mechanical issues are addressed concurrently. When supplementation is required, expressed human milk is preferred, followed by donor milk when available, with artificial substitutes used when necessary. Volume and frequency of supplementation should be individualized based on clinical indicators rather than predetermined schedules. Methods that preserve breastfeeding stimulation, such as supplemental feeding devices at the breast, paced alternative feeding techniques, or cup feeding, may reduce risk of nipple confusion and maintain oral skill development. Clear communication with families is essential to frame supplementation as a temporary medical support rather than a failure of breastfeeding. Documentation of supplementation indications and ongoing reassessment ensures timely return to exclusive breastfeeding when appropriate. Simultaneous protection of milk supply through pumping or hand expression is critical when direct feeding is insufficient. Abrupt or unnecessary supplementation may decrease breast stimulation and reduce long-term production. A structured plan that includes criteria for tapering supplementation supports gradual transition back to full breastfeeding once infant intake and growth stabilize.

Milk Expression: Hand Expression and Pumping

Milk expression is an essential technique for establishing, maintaining, or increasing milk supply when direct breastfeeding is not fully effective. Hand expression is particularly valuable in the early postpartum period when colostrum volumes are small and viscous. The technique involves rhythmic compression of the areolar tissue behind the nipple to stimulate milk flow without sliding fingers along the skin. Early and frequent hand expression within the first hour after birth enhances prolactin receptor development and improves long-term supply, especially when infants are preterm or separated. Mechanical pumping may be introduced when sustained separation occurs or when additional stimulation is needed. Effective pumping requires appropriate flange sizing to prevent nipple trauma and optimize milk removal. Pumping frequency should approximate normal feeding patterns, typically eight to twelve sessions per 24 hours in early lactation. Simultaneous double pumping may increase prolactin response and reduce total pumping time. Breast massage and compression during pumping can enhance yield by promoting additional let-down reflexes. Emotional relaxation techniques may improve oxytocin release and milk flow. Safe storage practices preserve milk quality, and education regarding cleaning of equipment reduces contamination risk. Mastery of expression techniques empowers families facing medical complications, employment separation, or relactation efforts and serves as a critical component of comprehensive lactation support.

Breast and Bottle Refusal Management

Breast refusal and bottle refusal represent feeding challenges that may arise from developmental changes, medical conditions, or environmental factors. Breast refusal may occur during periods of increased distractibility, teething discomfort, illness, or changes in milk flow. Infants may arch away, cry at the breast, or latch briefly before pulling off. Evaluation should assess milk ejection timing, latch comfort, and potential oversupply or low supply contributing to frustration. Skin-to-skin contact, feeding in a low-stimulation environment, and offering the breast during early hunger cues rather than distress may improve acceptance. Temporary breast refusal during illness often resolves spontaneously with supportive care. Bottle refusal, conversely, may occur when infants accustomed to direct breastfeeding resist artificial nipples due to differences in flow and oral mechanics. Gradual introduction of alternative feeding methods, paced techniques, and caregiver variation may facilitate acceptance. Timing attempts when the infant is calm but not overly hungry reduces stress. Avoiding forceful feeding prevents negative associations. In both scenarios, maintaining milk supply through regular expression is critical while feeding challenges are addressed. Parental reassurance is essential, as refusal behaviors can generate significant anxiety. Systematic assessment and patient, developmentally appropriate interventions typically restore effective feeding while preserving the breastfeeding relationship.

Chapter-7: Clinical Skills

Feeding Devices and Alternative Feeding Methods

Alternative feeding methods are used when direct breastfeeding is temporarily or partially ineffective, medically contraindicated, or developmentally inappropriate. The goal of any alternative feeding strategy is to ensure adequate nutrition while preserving oral development and protecting milk supply. Methods include cup feeding, spoon feeding, syringe feeding, finger feeding, and supplemental feeding devices that deliver milk at the breast. Selection depends on gestational age, medical stability, coordination of suck-swallow-breathe patterns, and duration of anticipated use. Cup feeding may be appropriate for term or late preterm infants with adequate swallowing reflexes, allowing the infant to lap milk without artificial nipple exposure. Syringe or finger feeding may be used for short-term supplementation while reinforcing sucking behavior. Supplemental feeding devices enable delivery of expressed milk through a small tube alongside the nipple, maintaining breast stimulation and reinforcing latch skills. Each method requires caregiver education to ensure safe pacing and minimize aspiration risk. Rapid flow or forced feeding can disrupt infant self-regulation and create aversive experiences. Careful assessment of infant fatigue, color changes, and swallowing patterns ensures safety. Alternative feeding should be accompanied by a clear plan for reassessment and transition back to exclusive breastfeeding when feasible. Maintaining maternal milk supply through consistent expression during periods of alternative feeding is critical. Proper instruction and follow-up reduce confusion and anxiety, supporting both adequate nutrition and long-term breastfeeding goals.

Pumps, Nipple Devices, and Equipment Use

Breast pumps and nipple devices are tools that require skilled guidance to ensure appropriate use and prevent complications. Pumps vary in mechanism, strength, and intended duration of use, and selection should align with clinical circumstances such as exclusive pumping, preterm birth, or temporary separation. Proper flange sizing is essential to avoid nipple trauma, optimize milk removal, and prevent discomfort. Incorrect sizing may lead to friction injury, reduced output, and compromised milk supply. Pump settings should balance adequate suction with comfort, beginning with stimulation mode to trigger let-down followed by expression mode once milk flow begins. Overly high suction does not increase yield and may damage tissue. Nipple shields are sometimes used to address latch difficulties, flat or inverted nipples, or infant oral coordination challenges. While shields may facilitate short-term feeding, they require monitoring to ensure adequate milk transfer and weight gain. Long-term unsupervised use may reduce breast stimulation if not properly managed. Pacifiers and artificial nipples should be introduced thoughtfully to minimize interference with established latch mechanics. Equipment hygiene, including proper cleaning and storage, prevents contamination and infection. Education regarding device assembly, maintenance, and safe transport of expressed milk enhances effectiveness. Competent instruction ensures that technological tools support rather than hinder lactation success.

Handling and Storage of Human Milk

Proper handling and storage of human milk preserve its nutritional and immunologic integrity while ensuring infant safety. Freshly expressed milk contains living cells, enzymes, and bioactive components that support immune function and gastrointestinal maturation. Clean expression techniques and sanitized storage containers minimize contamination risk. Milk may be stored at room temperature for limited periods depending on environmental conditions, with longer storage achievable under refrigeration or freezing. Temperature stability is critical, as repeated warming and cooling may degrade components and promote bacterial growth. When freezing, leaving space in containers allows for expansion. Thawing should occur gradually in the refrigerator or under warm running water rather than using high heat, which can damage protective factors. Once thawed, previously frozen milk should not be refrozen and should be used within recommended time frames. Gentle swirling rather than vigorous shaking helps reincorporate separated fat without excessive cellular disruption. For hospitalized or preterm infants, additional handling protocols may apply to ensure safety in vulnerable populations. Education of caregivers regarding labeling with dates and maintaining organized storage systems prevents waste and confusion. Safe transport of milk during travel or return to work requires insulated containers with appropriate cooling elements. Meticulous adherence to storage guidelines supports both infant health and efficient use of expressed milk.

Scale Use and Milk Transfer Measurement

Accurate measurement of milk transfer may be necessary when concerns arise regarding weight gain or feeding adequacy. Sensitive electronic scales capable of measuring small weight changes allow pre- and post-feed assessments to estimate milk intake during a single feeding session. The process involves weighing the infant immediately before and after feeding, with the difference in grams approximating milliliters consumed, given the similar density of human milk and water. Precision requires consistent clothing or diaper status to avoid measurement error. While useful in specific clinical scenarios, test weighing should not replace comprehensive feeding assessment or become routine in the absence of clinical concern. Overreliance on single feeding measurements may cause unnecessary anxiety, as intake naturally varies between sessions. Instead, trends over time provide more meaningful information. Proper scale calibration and staff training ensure reliability of results. Interpretation must consider infant age, feeding frequency, and overall growth patterns. When used appropriately, milk transfer measurement can guide decisions regarding supplementation, pumping frequency, or evaluation of latch effectiveness. Clear communication with families about the purpose and limitations of test weighing prevents misinterpretation. Skilled integration of objective data with clinical observation enhances decision-making while maintaining a supportive feeding environment.

Communication Technology and Virtual Care

Advancements in communication technology have expanded access to lactation support through telehealth and virtual consultation platforms. Virtual care allows real-time observation of feeding, positioning, and latch assessment when in-person visits are not feasible. Effective virtual consultation requires clear audio-visual setup, caregiver guidance in camera positioning, and privacy considerations. While tactile assessment is limited, skilled questioning and observation can identify many common challenges. Digital tools may facilitate sharing of weight logs, elimination patterns, and photographs of nipple trauma for evaluation. Virtual support is particularly valuable in rural or underserved areas and during public health emergencies when travel is restricted. However, clinicians must recognize limitations, including inability to perform hands-on oral assessments or measure weight directly. Establishing criteria for referral to in-person evaluation ensures safety when complex issues arise. Confidentiality and secure communication platforms are essential to protect personal health information. Virtual education sessions, support groups, and follow-up visits enhance continuity of care and may improve long-term breastfeeding outcomes. Technology should complement rather than replace comprehensive clinical judgment. With appropriate protocols, virtual lactation care expands accessibility while maintaining professional standards and individualized support.

Comprehensive Lactation Assessment

A comprehensive lactation assessment integrates maternal history, infant history, physical examination, feeding observation, and psychosocial context to form a complete clinical picture. Maternal assessment includes obstetric history, prior breastfeeding experience, medical conditions, medications, breast surgery, endocrine disorders, and postpartum recovery status. Breast examination may evaluate glandular development, nipple anatomy, evidence of trauma, engorgement, or infection. Infant assessment includes gestational age, birth weight, weight trajectory, elimination patterns, medical diagnoses, and neurologic tone. Direct observation of a feeding session provides critical information regarding positioning, latch depth, sucking rhythm, swallowing frequency, and maternal comfort. Evaluation extends beyond mechanics to include maternal confidence, support systems, and environmental stressors. A skilled clinician synthesizes subjective reports and objective findings to identify underlying causes of presenting concerns rather than addressing symptoms in isolation. Documentation should be clear, detailed, and clinically relevant, capturing both strengths and areas requiring intervention. Differential considerations may include supply issues, oral anatomical variations, hormonal influences, or behavioral factors. Reassessment over time is often necessary to evaluate response to interventions. Effective assessment is dynamic rather than static and requires critical thinking, pattern recognition, and evidence-based reasoning. By systematically integrating multiple data points, clinicians develop individualized care plans that support safe, effective, and sustainable feeding outcomes.

Clinical Reasoning and Care Planning

Clinical reasoning in lactation care involves analyzing assessment findings to prioritize problems, identify contributing factors, and design targeted interventions. Rather than applying standardized solutions, clinicians must adapt strategies to the unique physiologic and psychosocial characteristics of each dyad. Prioritization ensures that urgent concerns such as dehydration, excessive weight loss, or infection are addressed promptly while also creating space to manage longer-term goals such as improving latch comfort or transitioning away from supplementation. Care planning should be collaborative, incorporating parental goals, cultural values, and practical constraints. Clear, measurable objectives facilitate evaluation of progress, such as improving weight gain trajectory, reducing nipple pain, or increasing milk output over a defined period. Anticipatory guidance prepares families for expected developmental changes and potential challenges, reducing anxiety and promoting proactive management. Effective care plans also include criteria for follow-up and referral when indicated. Documentation of reasoning processes enhances continuity of care and supports interdisciplinary communication. Reflection on outcomes strengthens clinical expertise over time. Sound clinical reasoning integrates current evidence, physiologic principles, and compassionate understanding of family dynamics. This structured yet flexible approach ensures that interventions address root causes and support optimal feeding success.

Documentation and Professional Communication

Accurate documentation is a foundational clinical skill that supports patient safety, continuity of care, and professional accountability. Records should include relevant history, assessment findings, identified problems, interventions implemented, education provided, and plans for follow-up. Objective language enhances clarity and reduces ambiguity. Timely documentation ensures that other healthcare providers have access to current information, facilitating coordinated care. Communication extends beyond written records to include verbal discussions with interdisciplinary team members such as physicians, nurses, speech-language pathologists, and mental health professionals. Clear articulation of lactation-related findings promotes integrated management, particularly in complex cases involving medical or developmental conditions. Effective communication with families requires empathy, cultural sensitivity, and avoidance of jargon. Confirming understanding through teach-back methods enhances adherence and safety. Confidentiality and adherence to privacy regulations are essential components of ethical practice. Digital record systems require secure handling and appropriate access controls. Professional communication also includes advocacy when institutional policies or practices undermine breastfeeding support. Mastery of documentation and communication skills strengthens professional credibility and ensures that lactation care is recognized as an integral component of comprehensive healthcare.

Interdisciplinary Collaboration and Referral

Breastfeeding challenges often intersect with medical, surgical, psychological, and social domains, making interdisciplinary collaboration essential. Coordination with obstetric providers may be necessary for management of postpartum complications, endocrine disorders, or medication considerations. Pediatric collaboration is critical when addressing weight gain concerns, jaundice, prematurity, or congenital anomalies affecting feeding. Referral to speech-language pathologists or occupational therapists may support infants with oral motor dysfunction or coordination challenges. Mental health professionals play a vital role when maternal mood disorders or trauma histories influence feeding experiences. Social workers may assist families facing socioeconomic barriers that impede access to supplies or follow-up care. Effective collaboration requires mutual respect, clear role delineation, and timely information sharing. Understanding the scope and limitations of one's professional role ensures appropriate referral rather than attempting to manage conditions beyond expertise. Advocacy for breastfeeding-supportive practices within healthcare institutions strengthens systemic outcomes. Interdisciplinary teamwork enhances problem-solving capacity and ensures that families receive comprehensive, holistic care. Recognizing when referral is indicated demonstrates clinical maturity and commitment to patient-centered practice.

Quality Improvement, Ethics, and Professional Boundaries

Quality improvement in lactation care involves systematic evaluation of clinical outcomes, adherence to evidence-based guidelines, and implementation of strategies that enhance service effectiveness. Continuous professional development ensures that clinicians remain current with evolving research and recommendations. Ethical practice requires respect for parental autonomy, informed consent, and nondiscriminatory care regardless of feeding choices. Counseling should present evidence clearly without coercion, recognizing that families ultimately determine their feeding decisions. Professional boundaries protect both clinician and client, maintaining appropriate therapeutic relationships and avoiding dual roles that may compromise objectivity. Cultural humility and reflective practice support equitable care across diverse populations. Addressing implicit bias strengthens fairness and improves access to support. Documentation of adverse events and participation in peer review processes contribute to system-wide learning. Advocacy for policies that protect breastfeeding rights and access to care aligns with broader public health goals. Ethical dilemmas may arise when medical recommendations conflict with parental preferences; respectful dialogue and shared decision-making frameworks help navigate these situations. Commitment to quality improvement and ethical standards elevates clinical practice and reinforces trust in lactation professionals.

Chapter 8 – Practice Question and Answers

Questions (1-100)

Q1. Which reflex primarily ensures that a newborn can locate and latch onto the breast?
A. Palmar grasp reflex
B. Rooting reflex
C. Moro reflex
D. Stepping reflex

Q2. At approximately what age does an exclusively breastfed infant typically double their birth weight?
A. 2 months
B. 4 months
C. 6 months
D. 9 months

Q3. Which macronutrient in human milk contributes most to brain development during infancy?
A. Lactose
B. Protein
C. Long-chain polyunsaturated fatty acids
D. Minerals

Q4. What is the primary carbohydrate in human milk, serving as an important energy source for infants?
A. Glucose
B. Galactose
C. Lactose
D. Maltose

Q5. Which vitamin is lowest in concentration in human milk, potentially requiring supplementation?
A. Vitamin D
B. Vitamin C
C. Vitamin A
D. Vitamin E

Q6. Colostrum differs from mature milk primarily because it:
A. Has higher fat content
B. Contains less immunologic activity
C. Is rich in proteins and antibodies
D. Has lower mineral content

Q7. Which of the following best describes the composition of transitional milk?
A. High in immunoglobulins, low in fat
B. Increasing lactose and fat, decreasing protein
C. Constant composition after day one
D. Similar to colostrum throughout lactation

Q8. The World Health Organization recommends exclusive breastfeeding for:
A. 3 months
B. 4 months
C. 6 months
D. 12 months

Q9. Which growth chart standard is recommended by WHO for assessing exclusively breastfed infants globally?
A. CDC growth charts
B. Local percentile charts
C. WHO Child Growth Standards (2006)

D. Fenton preterm growth charts

Q10. Which human milk protein supports iron absorption in the infant gut?

A. Casein
B. Albumin
C. Lactoferrin
D. Lysozyme

Q11. Preterm milk differs from term milk primarily in its:

A. Lower protein concentration
B. Higher carbohydrate levels
C. Higher protein and immunologic components
D. Reduced fat-soluble vitamins

Q12. A mother's intake of which nutrient most directly influences DHA levels in her breast milk?

A. Protein
B. Omega-3 fatty acids
C. Calcium
D. Iron

Q13. What is the predominant immunoglobulin found in human milk?

A. IgG
B. IgA
C. IgM
D. IgE

Q14. Which factor most influences maternal milk volume?

A. Maternal diet
B. Breast size
C. Frequency and effectiveness of milk removal
D. Hormonal contraception use

Q15. Which maternal condition most strongly affects milk composition quality?

A. Mild dehydration
B. Severe malnutrition
C. Maternal anxiety
D. Sedentary lifestyle

Q16. What component of breast milk promotes the growth of beneficial intestinal bacteria in infants?

A. Lactose
B. Human milk oligosaccharides (HMOs)
C. Casein
D. Albumin

Q17. Which maternal factor most influences milk's immunologic properties?

A. Caloric intake
B. Parity
C. Exposure to local pathogens
D. Maternal age

Q18. Which trace mineral concentration is tightly regulated in human milk regardless of maternal intake?

A. Zinc
B. Iodine
C. Iron
D. Selenium

Q19. Which maternal hormone initiates milk secretion postpartum (lactogenesis II)?

A. Estrogen
B. Progesterone
C. Prolactin
D. Oxytocin

Q20. Which hormone primarily regulates milk ejection (let-down reflex)?
A. Prolactin
B. Cortisol
C. Oxytocin
D. Progesterone

Q21. Which hormone is primarily responsible for stimulating alveolar milk production?
A. Estrogen
B. Prolactin
C. Oxytocin
D. Thyroxine

Q22. During which stage of lactogenesis is milk secretion hormonally driven by declining progesterone levels?
A. Lactogenesis I
B. Lactogenesis II
C. Lactogenesis III
D. Galactopoiesis

Q23. Which endocrine feedback mechanism ensures milk production matches infant demand?
A. Positive feedback of oxytocin
B. Autocrine control via FIL protein
C. Negative feedback of prolactin
D. Adrenal cortisol modulation

Q24. Which nutrient in human milk is most critical for retinal development?
A. DHA
B. Vitamin A
C. Iron
D. Calcium

Q25. Oxytocin release during breastfeeding is stimulated by:
A. Breast fullness
B. Infant crying or suckling
C. Decreased estrogen
D. Maternal dehydration

Q26. Which maternal dietary component best enhances breast milk's vitamin A content?
A. Leafy greens
B. Citrus fruits
C. Carotenoid-rich vegetables
D. Whole grains

Q27. Which pituitary condition most likely results in agalactia postpartum?
A. Cushing's disease
B. Sheehan's syndrome
C. Prolactinoma
D. Hyperthyroidism

Q28. Why do preterm infants require higher protein concentration in expressed breast milk?
A. Reduced digestive enzyme efficiency
B. Increased metabolic and growth demands

C. Low fat absorption
D. Immature renal clearance
Q29. Which hormone promotes mammary ductal growth during pregnancy?
A. Prolactin
B. Estrogen
C. Oxytocin
D. Cortisol
Q30. Which mineral in human milk plays a crucial role in bone mineralization and muscle contraction?
A. Potassium
B. Sodium
C. Calcium
D. Magnesium
Q31. What role does cortisol play in lactation physiology?
A. Stimulates oxytocin secretion
B. Enhances milk ejection reflex
C. Supports mammary epithelial differentiation
D. Inhibits prolactin receptor formation
Q32. Which bioactive component of human milk protects against necrotizing enterocolitis in preterm infants?
A. Lactose
B. HMOs
C. Albumin
D. Vitamin C
Q33. What physiological change suppresses ovulation during exclusive breastfeeding?
A. Elevated estrogen
B. Reduced prolactin
C. High prolactin inhibiting GnRH secretion
D. Increased LH pulse frequency
Q34. Which complementary food introduction timing supports sustained growth and breastfeeding continuation?
A. 3 months
B. 4 months
C. 6 months
D. 9 months
Q35. What is the main role of oxytocin during milk ejection?
A. Stimulate alveolar synthesis
B. Contract myoepithelial cells
C. Increase blood supply
D. Decrease ductal resistance
Q36. Which factor most contributes to optimal infant gut microbiota establishment?
A. Early formula exposure
B. Breastfeeding exclusivity
C. Maternal antibiotic use
D. Cesarean delivery
Q37. Which endocrine organ malfunction can reduce prolactin levels and impair milk production?
A. Adrenal gland
B. Hypothalamus
C. Thyroid gland

D. Pancreas

Q38. Which fatty acid ratio in human milk promotes anti-inflammatory effects in infants?

A. Omega-6:Omega-3 ratio of 1:1
B. Omega-6:Omega-3 ratio of 5–10:1
C. Omega-6 dominance (>20:1)
D. No measurable ratio impact

Q39. Which hormone's pulsatile secretion maintains prolactin release during lactation?

A. Dopamine
B. GnRH
C. TRH
D. Oxytocin

Q40. Which metabolic adaptation ensures consistent milk fat synthesis during maternal fasting periods?

A. Increased glucose uptake by mammary cells
B. Enhanced mobilization of maternal adipose stores
C. Reduced prolactin sensitivity
D. Decreased alveolar lipid synthesis

Q41. Which factor best reflects adequate breastfeeding in a newborn during the first week?

A. Crying after every feed
B. Six or more wet diapers daily by day 5
C. Weight loss exceeding 10%
D. Passing no stools by day 3

Q42. Which maternal micronutrient deficiency most likely results in low infant iodine levels?

A. Iron
B. Zinc
C. Iodine
D. Vitamin C

Q43. Which process maintains ongoing lactation beyond the early postpartum period?

A. Hormonal prolactin surge only
B. Autocrine control by milk removal
C. Continuous oxytocin release
D. Increasing estrogen feedback

Q44. Which feeding behavior indicates readiness for complementary foods?

A. Tongue-thrust reflex persists
B. Head and neck control established
C. Exclusive milk preference
D. Inability to sit unsupported

Q45. What is the physiological role of progesterone in breast development during pregnancy?

A. Stimulates ductal growth
B. Promotes alveolar cell differentiation
C. Triggers oxytocin release
D. Inhibits prolactin receptor formation

Q46. Which maternal dietary pattern enhances vitamin B12 content in breast milk?

A. Strict vegan diet
B. Balanced omnivorous intake
C. High-fiber vegetarian diet
D. Gluten-free diet

Q47. Which factor contributes most to slower growth velocity in exclusively breastfed infants after six months?

A. Lower protein density of breast milk
B. Decreasing maternal hydration
C. Reduced feeding frequency
D. Iron deficiency

Q48. Which maternal hormone rises during pregnancy but inhibits milk secretion until birth?
A. Oxytocin
B. Estrogen
C. Progesterone
D. Prolactin

Q49. Which indicator best reflects normal infant feeding frequency in the first month?
A. Every 1–2 hours
B. Every 3–4 hours
C. Every 6 hours
D. Once or twice daily

Q50. Which factor most directly stimulates prolactin release during breastfeeding?
A. Suckling-induced neural signals to hypothalamus
B. Drop in estrogen and progesterone
C. Elevated oxytocin concentration
D. Increased dopamine secretion

Q51. Which type of infant stool indicates effective milk digestion and absorption in a breastfed baby?
A. Pale and pasty
B. Green and watery
C. Yellow, seedy, and soft
D. Hard and formed

Q52. Which hormone supports mammary gland differentiation alongside prolactin and cortisol?
A. Thyroxine
B. Growth hormone
C. Insulin
D. Oxytocin

Q53. Which maternal illness most compromises vitamin A content in breast milk?
A. Mild hypothyroidism
B. Severe protein-calorie malnutrition
C. Iron-deficiency anemia
D. Postpartum depression

Q54. Which structure synthesizes and secretes prolactin?
A. Hypothalamus
B. Anterior pituitary
C. Posterior pituitary
D. Mammary alveoli

Q55. How does maternal obesity influence breastfeeding initiation?
A. Enhances milk flow rate
B. Delays lactogenesis II
C. Increases prolactin sensitivity
D. Shortens suckling duration

Q56. Which factor most accurately predicts future breastfeeding success?
A. Early skin-to-skin contact post-birth
B. Birth weight percentile
C. Maternal age

D. Mode of delivery
Q57. What effect does dopamine have on prolactin release during lactation?
A. Stimulates release
B. Inhibits secretion
C. Neutral effect
D. Increases oxytocin sensitivity
Q58. Which maternal factor increases lactose concentration in milk?
A. Increased dietary calcium
B. Frequent and complete breast emptying
C. High-protein intake
D. Elevated cortisol
Q59. Which maternal gland is crucial for maintaining basal metabolic rate during lactation?
A. Adrenal
B. Thyroid
C. Pituitary
D. Pancreas
Q60. Which factor ensures optimal calcium absorption in breastfeeding infants?
A. High lactose content of milk
B. Maternal calcium supplementation
C. Iron-rich complementary foods
D. Reduced phosphorus content
Q61. Which component of breast milk promotes intestinal maturation and mucosal protection?
A. Lactose
B. Epidermal growth factor (EGF)
C. Casein
D. Vitamin D
Q62. Which event triggers the switch from endocrine to autocrine control of milk production?
A. Placental delivery
B. Infant's first latch
C. Engorgement phase resolution
D. Onset of mature milk flow
Q63. Which factor distinguishes foremilk from hindmilk during a single feed?
A. Protein concentration
B. Fat content
C. Lactose levels
D. Vitamin A content
Q64. Which neurotransmitter primarily inhibits prolactin secretion in the hypothalamus?
A. GABA
B. Serotonin
C. Dopamine
D. Acetylcholine
Q65. Which maternal health condition most risks delayed lactogenesis II?
A. Gestational diabetes
B. Hypertension
C. Iron deficiency
D. Thyroid nodules
Q66. What effect does stress have on oxytocin-mediated milk ejection?
A. Enhances reflex

B. Temporarily inhibits release
C. Reduces milk synthesis
D. Permanently decreases prolactin

Q67. Which factor ensures sufficient iron stores in full-term infants?
A. Late umbilical cord clamping
B. Early complementary feeding
C. Maternal calcium intake
D. Frequent urination

Q68. Which endocrine disorder may cause low milk supply despite adequate glandular tissue?
A. Hyperprolactinemia
B. Hypothyroidism
C. Hyperthyroidism
D. Adrenal insufficiency

Q69. Which maternal macronutrient primarily determines total milk energy content?
A. Protein
B. Fat
C. Carbohydrate
D. Mineral

Q70. What is the role of oxytocin in maternal-infant bonding?
A. Inhibits cortisol release
B. Enhances stress response
C. Promotes emotional bonding and calmness
D. Increases maternal prolactin levels

Q71. Which infant population benefits most from donor human milk?
A. Term infants with poor latch
B. Preterm or very low birthweight infants
C. Infants of diabetic mothers
D. Infants with reflux

Q72. Which maternal hormone primarily drives breast alveolar cell differentiation during pregnancy?
A. Estrogen
B. Progesterone
C. Prolactin
D. Cortisol

Q73. Which milk component supports brain myelination in infants?
A. Lactose
B. DHA
C. Calcium
D. Albumin

Q74. What mechanism prevents milk leakage between feedings?
A. Sphincter contraction at nipple base
B. Alveolar fat thickening
C. Oxytocin inhibition during rest
D. Tight junction closure in mammary epithelium

Q75. Which growth pattern is normal for breastfed infants in the first six months?
A. Rapid linear gain, then plateau
B. Gradual continuous gain with slower later velocity
C. Consistent high-weight trajectory beyond 95th percentile
D. Decline below WHO median by 3 months

Q76. Which hormone's receptor upregulation marks transition to active milk synthesis postpartum?
A. Progesterone
B. Prolactin
C. Cortisol
D. Insulin
Q77. Which WHO chart parameter adjusts for gestational age in preterm infants?
A. Chronological age only
B. Corrected age
C. Weight-for-length z-score
D. BMI-for-age percentile
Q78. Which pathway integrates neuroendocrine signaling between suckling and oxytocin release?
A. Hypothalamic-pituitary-gonadal
B. Hypothalamic-pituitary-adrenal
C. Hypothalamic-pituitary-neurohypophyseal
D. Sympathetic-adrenal medullary
Q79. Which maternal nutrient most affects milk's antioxidant capacity?
A. Vitamin E
B. Vitamin D
C. Iron
D. Selenium
Q80. Which physiological mechanism ensures synchronized milk ejection from both breasts?
A. Local nerve reflexes
B. Systemic oxytocin release
C. Alternate nipple stimulation
D. Prolactin rebound
Q81. Which factor contributes most to establishing early milk supply?
A. Delayed initiation of breastfeeding
B. Frequent, on-demand feeding
C. Nighttime feeding avoidance
D. Scheduled feeding every 4 hours
Q82. What is the role of cortisol during lactogenesis I?
A. Inhibits prolactin receptor formation
B. Promotes mammary epithelial differentiation
C. Reduces milk fat synthesis
D. Suppresses oxytocin release
Q83. Which complementary feeding principle aligns with WHO guidelines?
A. Introduce solids at 4 months for rapid growth
B. Begin at 6 months while maintaining breastfeeding
C. Provide cow's milk as early calcium source
D. Delay solids until 9 months
Q84. Which hypothalamic nucleus regulates oxytocin synthesis?
A. Suprachiasmatic nucleus
B. Paraventricular nucleus
C. Arcuate nucleus
D. Ventromedial nucleus
Q85. Which human milk property provides protection against gastrointestinal infections?
A. High sodium concentration
B. Presence of secretory IgA

C. Elevated lactose
D. Low osmolality

Q86. Which hormone increases mammary blood flow during lactation?
A. Oxytocin
B. Estrogen
C. Prolactin
D. Cortisol

Q87. Which breast milk component supports intestinal immune development by shaping gut flora?
A. Lactose
B. HMOs
C. Casein
D. Vitamin D

Q88. Which feedback mechanism regulates prolactin release post-suckling?
A. Positive oxytocin reinforcement
B. Dopaminergic inhibition restoration
C. Continuous hypothalamic stimulation
D. Estrogen pulse suppression

Q89. Which maternal behavior promotes effective milk transfer?
A. Rigid feeding schedule
B. Responsive feeding based on infant cues
C. Limiting feed duration to 10 minutes
D. Offering one breast per day

Q90. Which hormone promotes alveolar milk lipid synthesis?
A. Cortisol
B. Insulin
C. Estrogen
D. Prolactin

Q91. Which maternal vitamin deficiency is most likely to cause rickets in an exclusively breastfed infant?
A. Vitamin K
B. Vitamin E
C. Vitamin D
D. Vitamin A

Q92. Which receptor type mediates oxytocin's action on myoepithelial cells?
A. GABA receptor
B. G-protein–coupled receptor
C. Ionotropic calcium channel
D. Nuclear receptor

Q93. Which breastfeeding position best promotes airway patency and latch stability in newborns?
A. Cradle hold
B. Football hold
C. Side-lying hold
D. Upright seated hold

Q94. Which maternal endocrine response supports relaxation during feeding?
A. Elevated cortisol
B. Decreased oxytocin
C. Oxytocin-induced parasympathetic activation
D. Increased sympathetic tone

Q95. Which biochemical characteristic differentiates human milk protein from cow's milk protein?

A. Higher casein proportion
B. Greater whey dominance
C. Lack of immunoglobulins
D. Identical amino acid profile

Q96. Which glandular structure stores oxytocin before release?
A. Anterior pituitary
B. Posterior pituitary
C. Adrenal medulla
D. Thyroid follicle

Q97. What determines variability in breast milk flavor?
A. Maternal fluid intake
B. Maternal diet composition
C. Milk storage duration
D. Infant age

Q98. Which physiological response is impaired by high dopamine levels?
A. Oxytocin secretion
B. Cortisol metabolism
C. Estrogen synthesis
D. Prolactin release

Q99. What is the typical protein ratio (whey:casein) in mature human milk?
A. 20:80
B. 60:40
C. 80:20
D. 50:50

Q100. Which maternal factor enhances oxytocin secretion during breastfeeding?
A. Anxiety
B. Infant cry and tactile stimulation
C. Sleep deprivation
D. Maternal dehydration

Answer key and Explanation (1-100)

Q1. Answer: B

Explanation: The rooting reflex enables an infant to turn toward touch near the mouth, facilitating latching. This reflex supports early feeding behavior by aligning oral orientation with the nipple. Other reflexes, such as palmar grasp or Moro, do not directly influence breastfeeding mechanics.

Q2. Answer: C

Explanation: Most exclusively breastfed infants double their birth weight by about six months. This reflects adequate nutritional intake and growth per WHO standards. While formula-fed infants may gain weight faster, the growth trajectory for breastfed infants is physiologically normal and healthful.

Q3. Answer: C

Explanation: Long-chain polyunsaturated fatty acids, particularly DHA and ARA, are critical for neuronal and retinal development. They influence synaptic formation and visual acuity. Although lactose provides energy, fats are more directly linked to neurodevelopmental outcomes.

Q4. Answer: C

Explanation: Lactose constitutes about 7% of human milk and is the key carbohydrate providing energy for infant metabolism and aiding calcium absorption. Glucose and galactose are its monomers, but lactose's unique osmotic properties drive milk volume and hydration balance.

Q5. Answer: A

Explanation: Human milk contains low vitamin D levels, insufficient to meet infant requirements without sunlight exposure or supplementation. While vitamins A and E are fat-soluble and present in reasonable amounts, vitamin D depends on maternal status and UV exposure.

Q6. Answer: C

Explanation: Colostrum is protein- and antibody-rich, providing immunologic protection through secretory IgA. It supports intestinal maturation and passive immunity. Fat content increases in mature milk as energy needs rise; colostrum emphasizes protection over caloric density.

Q7. Answer: B

Explanation: Transitional milk (days 5–14) shows rising lactose and fat while protein levels decline. This supports rapid infant growth and expanding energy demands. The transition bridges colostrum's protective phase to mature milk's nutritive function.

Q8. Answer: C

Explanation: Exclusive breastfeeding for six months ensures optimal nutrition and immune protection. Introducing complementary foods earlier may reduce milk intake and increase infection risk. Continued breastfeeding alongside solid foods is advised up to two years or beyond.

Q9. Answer: C

Explanation: WHO 2006 Growth Standards are based on optimally nourished, breastfed infants worldwide, reflecting ideal growth patterns. CDC charts, derived largely from formula-fed cohorts, can misrepresent normal breastfed growth as slower or inadequate.

Q10. Answer: C

Explanation: Lactoferrin binds iron, preventing pathogenic bacterial growth and facilitating iron absorption. It plays a dual role in immunity and nutrition. Casein aids in calcium metabolism, while lysozyme serves antimicrobial functions without influencing iron uptake.

Q11. Answer: C

Explanation: Preterm milk contains higher protein, nitrogen, and immune factors to meet the increased metabolic and developmental needs of preterm infants. It compensates for immaturity of organ systems, promoting neurodevelopment and infection defense.

Q12. Answer: B

Explanation: Maternal omega-3 fatty acid consumption, especially from marine sources, raises DHA in milk, essential for neural and visual development. Protein, calcium, and iron contribute to general nutrition but do not alter DHA concentration significantly.

Q13. Answer: B

Explanation: Secretory IgA provides mucosal defense by coating infant gut linings and neutralizing pathogens. It prevents adherence of microbes without causing inflammation. IgG dominates systemic immunity, not localized mucosal protection.

Q14. Answer: C

Explanation: Frequent and complete milk removal maintains prolactin response and alveolar emptying, ensuring sustained production. While nutrition supports health, mechanical stimulation regulates supply-demand physiology. Hormonal contraception may affect volume but less consistently.

Q15. Answer: B

Explanation: Severe malnutrition may lower key micronutrients and energy content in milk, affecting infant growth. Mild dehydration or stress rarely alters composition significantly. The mammary gland protects nutrient transfer efficiency even under moderate maternal strain.

Q16. Answer: B

Explanation: HMOs act as prebiotics, fostering Bifidobacteria colonization and inhibiting pathogen binding. They contribute to gut maturation and immune modulation. Unlike lactose, HMOs are indigestible but biologically active in shaping intestinal microbiota.

Q17. Answer: C

Explanation: Antibody specificity in milk reflects maternal antigen exposure, transferring localized immunity to the infant. Caloric intake affects volume, not immune composition. The adaptive immune system tailors sIgA responses to current environmental pathogens.

Q18. Answer: C

Explanation: Iron concentration in human milk remains stable due to tight homeostatic control, protecting infants from overload and deficiency. Zinc and iodine reflect maternal status more closely. This ensures safe and balanced early hematologic development.

Q19. Answer: C

Explanation: Prolactin triggers milk synthesis once progesterone levels fall after delivery. Estrogen and progesterone inhibit secretion during pregnancy. Oxytocin instead mediates milk ejection, not synthesis. This hormonal shift defines the onset of true lactation.

Q20. Answer: C

Explanation: Oxytocin released from the posterior pituitary causes myoepithelial cell contraction, propelling milk through ducts during suckling. Prolactin maintains milk synthesis, while cortisol supports metabolism. Progesterone declines post-birth, allowing lactation onset.

Q21. Answer: B

Explanation: Prolactin from the anterior pituitary stimulates alveolar cells to synthesize milk. It acts in response to nipple stimulation, maintaining lactation through feedback inhibition balance. Estrogen and oxytocin support structural and ejection roles, respectively.

Q22. Answer: B

Explanation: Lactogenesis II begins after placental delivery when progesterone drops, removing inhibition on prolactin receptors. This enables copious milk secretion. Earlier stages involve alveolar differentiation, while galactopoiesis maintains established lactation.

Q23. Answer: B

Explanation: The Feedback Inhibitor of Lactation (FIL) protein regulates secretion locally; accumulated milk suppresses synthesis. This autocrine loop balances supply with removal frequency. Hormones establish production, but FIL fine-tunes daily milk volume.

Q24. Answer: A

Explanation: DHA supports retinal photoreceptor growth and visual acuity maturation. It accumulates rapidly during late gestation and early infancy. Vitamin A contributes to general ocular health, but DHA directly influences neural retina development.

Q25. Answer: B

Explanation: Nipple stimulation by suckling or infant cues triggers oxytocin release from the posterior pituitary. This promotes milk ejection via myoepithelial contraction. Emotional bonding also enhances oxytocin reflex through sensory integration pathways.

Q26. Answer: C

Explanation: Carotenoids from orange and yellow vegetables convert to retinol, enriching milk's vitamin A. This supports epithelial and immune development. While leafy greens provide folate, they have less impact on retinoid concentration in milk.

Q27. Answer: B

Explanation: Sheehan's syndrome, caused by pituitary infarction from postpartum hemorrhage, destroys prolactin-secreting cells leading to agalactia. Prolactinoma causes hypersecretion, not deficiency. Cushing's and thyroid disorders have secondary, lesser effects.

Q28. Answer: B

Explanation: Preterm infants grow faster relative to body mass and need additional amino acids for organ development. Enhanced protein concentration supports tissue repair and nitrogen balance. Digestion and renal issues exist but are secondary concerns.

Q29. Answer: B

Explanation: Estrogen stimulates ductal proliferation and vascularization, establishing the structural network for milk transport. Progesterone aids alveolar development, while prolactin primes secretory cells. Oxytocin acts postpartum for milk ejection, not growth.

Q30. Answer: C

Explanation: Calcium supports skeletal growth and neuromuscular function. Its bioavailability in human milk surpasses that in cow's milk due to balanced phosphorus ratios. Proper intake prevents hypocalcemia and fosters strong bone matrix formation.

Q31. Answer: C

Explanation: Cortisol facilitates mammary gland differentiation and metabolic readiness for milk synthesis. It interacts with prolactin during lactogenesis I. Though a stress hormone, physiologic cortisol levels are essential for functional secretory activation.

Q32. Answer: B

Explanation: Human milk oligosaccharides (HMOs) enhance gut integrity, inhibit pathogen adhesion, and reduce inflammation—key in preventing NEC. Their prebiotic effect supports beneficial microbiota balance crucial for immature preterm intestines.

Q33. Answer: C

Explanation: Sustained prolactin levels inhibit hypothalamic GnRH release, preventing LH surges and ovulation. This forms the physiologic basis of lactational amenorrhea. Once breastfeeding frequency drops, prolactin decreases, restoring fertility cycles.

Q34. Answer: C

Explanation: Complementary feeding at six months aligns with nutrient depletion of exclusive milk diets, ensuring balanced energy and micronutrient intake while maintaining breastfeeding benefits. Earlier introduction risks infection and reduced lactation duration.

Q35. Answer: B

Explanation: Oxytocin causes myoepithelial cells surrounding alveoli to contract, propelling milk toward ducts and nipple. This ejection reflex is triggered by suckling or emotional stimuli, ensuring efficient feeding cycles.

Q36. Answer: B

Explanation: Exclusive breastfeeding introduces beneficial bacteria and HMOs promoting microbiome stability. Formula exposure or maternal antibiotic use disrupts microbial balance. Early breastfeeding supports immune programming and nutrient absorption.

Q37. Answer: B

Explanation: The hypothalamus controls prolactin via dopamine inhibition. Damage or dysfunction may disturb regulatory balance, suppressing prolactin and thus lactation. Thyroid and adrenal hormones support metabolism but do not directly regulate prolactin synthesis.

Q38. Answer: B

Explanation: A balanced omega-6:omega-3 ratio (5–10:1) supports optimal inflammation control and neural development. Excess omega-6 intake reduces DHA availability and may impair immunoregulation in early infancy.

Q39. Answer: C

Explanation: Thyrotropin-releasing hormone (TRH) indirectly promotes prolactin release, especially when suckling stimuli persist. Dopamine inhibits prolactin, while oxytocin mediates ejection rather than synthesis. This interplay stabilizes milk output under neuroendocrine control.

Q40. Answer: B

Explanation: During fasting, maternal adipose tissue releases fatty acids mobilized for milk fat synthesis. This maintains infant nutrition even when caloric intake fluctuates. The mammary gland prioritizes milk production through adaptive energy partitioning.

Q41. Answer: B

Explanation: At least six wet diapers per day by day five indicates effective intake and hydration. Early weight loss under 10% is acceptable, but ongoing loss signals feeding issues. Regular stooling complements hydration as evidence of successful breastfeeding.

Q42. Answer: C

Explanation: Iodine deficiency reduces maternal thyroxine synthesis, lowering iodine transfer into milk. This can impair infant thyroid development. Unlike iron or zinc, iodine is not tightly regulated in milk and depends on maternal dietary intake.

Q43. Answer: B

Explanation: Galactopoiesis relies on local regulation through milk removal frequency. Prolactin initiates secretion, but ongoing supply is sustained by demand-driven emptying, ensuring homeostatic production proportional to infant needs.

Q44. Answer: B

Explanation: Head and neck control combined with diminished tongue-thrust reflex indicates oral motor readiness for solids. Introduction before developmental readiness can increase aspiration risk and disrupt breastfeeding.

Q45. Answer: B

Explanation: Progesterone promotes alveolar-lobular differentiation, preparing for milk synthesis. It balances estrogen's ductal effects to create functional secretory units. Inhibition of lactation persists until progesterone withdrawal post-delivery.

Q46. Answer: B

Explanation: A balanced omnivorous diet provides sufficient animal-derived cobalamin to enrich milk B12 levels. Strict vegan diets risk deficiency unless supplemented. Infant B12 deficiency can cause anemia and neurological impairment if maternal intake is inadequate.

Q47. Answer: A

Explanation: The natural decline in protein concentration limits caloric density, signaling readiness for complementary feeding. It represents a physiologic transition rather than deficiency. Adequate weaning foods correct the energy gap to maintain growth.

Q48. Answer: C

Explanation: Progesterone suppresses lactation despite high prolactin levels during pregnancy. Once the placenta is delivered, progesterone levels drop, allowing prolactin receptors to activate and initiate milk secretion (lactogenesis II).

Q49. Answer: B

Explanation: Newborns feed 8–12 times per day, typically every 2–3 hours, supporting steady milk production and growth. Longer intervals may indicate poor latch or inadequate stimulation affecting supply-demand balance.

Q50. Answer: A

Explanation: Suckling sends afferent impulses to the hypothalamus, inhibiting dopamine (prolactin-inhibiting factor), thereby stimulating prolactin secretion. This feedback maintains synthesis proportional to infant demand and ensures milk production stability.

Q51. Answer: C

Explanation: Yellow, seedy, soft stools reflect good fat digestion and nutrient absorption in breastfed infants. Hard stools suggest dehydration or formula feeding, while green watery stools may indicate foremilk imbalance or mild infection.

Q52. Answer: C

Explanation: Insulin promotes mammary epithelial cell growth and nutrient uptake required for milk synthesis. It works synergistically with cortisol and prolactin. Thyroxine influences metabolism indirectly but doesn't initiate glandular differentiation.

Q53. Answer: B

Explanation: Severe protein-calorie malnutrition reduces fat-soluble vitamin levels including vitamin A. Energy deprivation affects retinol storage and secretion. Other conditions minimally impact fat-soluble vitamin transfer unless accompanied by nutritional deficits.

Q54. Answer: B

Explanation: The anterior pituitary's lactotroph cells produce prolactin. Its release is regulated by hypothalamic dopamine inhibition. The posterior pituitary releases oxytocin, responsible for milk ejection rather than synthesis.

Q55. Answer: B

Explanation: Obesity is associated with delayed onset of copious milk production due to hormonal dysregulation and inflammatory mediators affecting prolactin response. Supportive interventions help maintain early stimulation and establish supply.

Q56. Answer: A

Explanation: Early skin-to-skin contact promotes oxytocin release, warmth regulation, and instinctive suckling behaviors, fostering immediate latch success and sustained lactation. It outweighs demographic or delivery mode influences.

Q57. Answer: B

Explanation: Dopamine from the hypothalamus acts as prolactin-inhibiting factor. Suckling suppresses dopamine, allowing prolactin release for milk synthesis. This inverse relationship ensures lactation occurs only with regular feeding stimulation.

Q58. Answer: B

Explanation: Frequent milk removal maintains lactose synthesis via osmotic regulation within alveoli. This promotes fluid secretion and milk volume consistency. Nutrient composition changes little with diet except during extreme malnutrition.

Q59. Answer: B

Explanation: The thyroid gland enhances metabolism and energy conversion, meeting the high caloric demand of milk synthesis. Hypothyroidism can impair lactation efficiency and milk output through reduced metabolic signaling.

Q60. Answer: A

Explanation: Lactose enhances calcium solubility and absorption efficiency in the infant intestine. Human milk's calcium-phosphorus ratio supports skeletal mineralization. Supplementation is rarely necessary with exclusive breastfeeding.

Q61. Answer: B

Explanation: EGF stimulates epithelial cell growth and repair, aiding gut barrier maturation. It reduces intestinal permeability, protecting against infection and allergy. Other nutrients support growth but do not directly drive epithelial development.

Q62. Answer: D

Explanation: Once mature milk flow is established, local feedback replaces systemic hormonal control. The autocrine phase maintains supply through milk removal signals. Endocrine dominance persists only during colostrum and early transitional phases.

Q63. Answer: B

Explanation: Hindmilk contains higher fat concentration, providing energy density for satiety. Foremilk is thinner, primarily hydrating and carbohydrate-rich. Complete breast emptying ensures balanced nutrient intake per feeding cycle.

Q64. Answer: C

Explanation: Dopamine acts as prolactin-inhibiting factor, tonically suppressing prolactin release. Suckling reduces dopamine output, allowing lactation. Other neurotransmitters may indirectly influence mood or reflexes but not primary prolactin control.

Q65. Answer: A

Explanation: Gestational diabetes interferes with insulin sensitivity, delaying lactogenesis II through hormonal dysregulation. Insulin plays a key metabolic role in mammary gland activation. Support and early stimulation mitigate delay effects.

Q66. Answer: B

Explanation: Stress elevates catecholamines that block oxytocin release from the posterior pituitary, impairing let-down reflex. This is transient and reversible with relaxation or skin-to-skin contact. Milk synthesis remains unaffected hormonally.

Q67. Answer: A

Explanation: Delayed cord clamping increases neonatal blood volume and iron stores, reducing anemia risk. Full-term infants maintain iron sufficiency for about six months, supported by breast milk bioavailability.

Q68. Answer: B

Explanation: Hypothyroidism reduces metabolic drive and prolactin receptor sensitivity, leading to low milk volume. Restoring thyroid hormones improves production. Hyperprolactinemia may paradoxically suppress gonadotropins but not lactation.

Q69. Answer: B

Explanation: Fat contributes the majority of milk energy, varying with maternal diet and stage of feeding. Its concentration rises through feeding, meeting infant energy needs. Carbohydrates provide volume but less caloric density.

Q70. Answer: C

Explanation: Oxytocin promotes feelings of calm, bonding, and trust through limbic activation during feeding. It strengthens emotional connection and maternal caregiving behaviors. Prolactin supports nurturing but not direct emotional bonding.

Q71. Answer: B

Explanation: Donor milk provides immunologic protection and optimal nutrition for preterm or VLBW infants, lowering NEC and infection risks. Formula use in this group increases morbidity despite caloric equivalence.

Q72. Answer: C

Explanation: Prolactin facilitates alveolar secretory cell differentiation in concert with progesterone and cortisol. Estrogen supports ductal growth, while cortisol ensures metabolic preparation for milk synthesis.

Q73. Answer: B

Explanation: DHA contributes to neural membrane integrity and myelination, optimizing cognitive and visual development. Adequate maternal intake of omega-3 sources enhances infant neurodevelopmental outcomes.

Q74. Answer: D

Explanation: Tight junctions between mammary epithelial cells seal milk within alveoli between feedings. Disruption causes leakage or engorgement. Oxytocin acts transiently only during feeding, not as a continuous sealant.

Q75. Answer: B

Explanation: Breastfed infants show steady growth, with slower velocity after three months. This reflects physiologic energy utilization, not undernutrition. WHO charts represent breastfed growth as normative standard.

Q76. Answer: B

Explanation: Prolactin receptor upregulation follows progesterone withdrawal, initiating lactogenesis II. This enhances secretory activity in alveolar cells. Cortisol and insulin assist metabolically but are not the primary trigger.

Q77. Answer: B

Explanation: Corrected age accounts for gestational weeks missed at birth, aligning assessment with developmental stage. This avoids misclassification of growth delay in preterm infants when plotting on WHO growth standards.

Q78. Answer: C

Explanation: The hypothalamic-pituitary-neurohypophyseal axis conducts suckling-induced neural impulses to the posterior pituitary, releasing oxytocin. This enables coordinated milk ejection. Other axes regulate stress or reproductive hormones, not lactation reflexes.

Q79. Answer: A

Explanation: Vitamin E, a lipid-soluble antioxidant, protects polyunsaturated fatty acids in milk from oxidation. Its concentration reflects maternal dietary fat intake and supports infant oxidative defense mechanisms.

Q80. Answer: B

Explanation: Oxytocin acts systemically via bloodstream, contracting myoepithelial cells in both breasts simultaneously. Local control affects production, but ejection depends on circulating hormone release ensuring bilateral let-down.

Q81. Answer: B

Explanation: Frequent, on-demand feeding promotes continuous prolactin stimulation and oxytocin release, optimizing supply establishment. Scheduled or delayed feeding disrupts hormonal cues and reduces milk production efficiency.

Q82. Answer: B

Explanation: Cortisol synergizes with prolactin and insulin to differentiate mammary epithelial cells before birth. It prepares the gland for secretion, supporting enzymatic readiness without triggering active milk synthesis prematurely.

Q83. Answer: B

Explanation: WHO recommends exclusive breastfeeding for six months, followed by nutrient-rich complementary foods while continuing breastfeeding to two years or more. This supports sustained nutrition and immune benefits.

Q84. Answer: B

Explanation: The paraventricular and supraoptic nuclei synthesize oxytocin, which is transported to the posterior pituitary for release. This neuroendocrine pathway links nipple stimulation with milk ejection and bonding reflexes.

Q85. Answer: B

Explanation: Secretory IgA coats mucosal surfaces, preventing pathogen adherence and infection. It forms part of the infant's passive immune defense. Other components contribute nutritionally but not directly to mucosal immunity.

Q86. Answer: C

Explanation: Prolactin enhances mammary blood flow to supply substrates for milk synthesis. Its action supports nutrient transfer and alveolar metabolism. Oxytocin controls ejection, while estrogen maintains ductal health postpartum.

Q87. Answer: B

Explanation: Human milk oligosaccharides (HMOs) selectively nourish beneficial bacteria like Bifidobacteria, fostering immune maturation. They also prevent pathogen adhesion to the intestinal lining, reducing infection risk.

Q88. Answer: B

Explanation: After feeding, dopamine secretion resumes, suppressing prolactin release until the next suckling episode. This prevents unnecessary milk synthesis between feeds and maintains endocrine balance.

Q89. Answer: B

Explanation: Feeding responsively to infant hunger cues enhances latch, oxytocin reflex, and milk ejection. Strict schedules reduce stimulation and disrupt hormonal rhythm essential for milk supply maintenance.

Q90. Answer: D

Explanation: Prolactin activates lipogenic enzymes in mammary epithelial cells, producing triglycerides for milk fat. Cortisol aids in energy mobilization, while insulin provides substrate availability for biosynthesis.

Q91. Answer: C

Explanation: Low maternal vitamin D results in reduced milk levels, predisposing infants to rickets. Supplementation or sunlight exposure is essential to maintain bone mineralization and calcium balance.

Q92. Answer: B

Explanation: Oxytocin binds to G-protein–coupled receptors on myoepithelial cells, triggering intracellular calcium release and contraction. This signaling enables coordinated milk ejection without direct metabolic effect.

Q93. Answer: B

Explanation: The football hold supports infant head and neck alignment, optimizing airway patency and latch control—especially useful for post-cesarean mothers or those with large breasts.

Q94. Answer: C

Explanation: Oxytocin release stimulates parasympathetic pathways, promoting calmness and bonding during feeding. This neuroendocrine effect counters stress responses and enhances let-down efficiency.

Q95. Answer: B

Explanation: Human milk is whey-dominant, offering easier digestibility and bioavailability of immunoglobulins and enzymes. Cow's milk is casein-rich, forming firmer curds that are less suited for immature infant digestion.

Q96. Answer: B

Explanation: The posterior pituitary (neurohypophysis) stores and releases oxytocin produced by hypothalamic neurons. Release occurs through neural impulses triggered by nipple stimulation.

Q97. Answer: B

Explanation: Volatile compounds from maternal diet, such as garlic or spices, transfer to milk, subtly influencing flavor. This exposure promotes later dietary acceptance and sensory familiarity for the infant.

Q98. Answer: D

Explanation: Elevated dopamine suppresses prolactin secretion, leading to reduced milk synthesis. Dopamine antagonists like metoclopramide can increase prolactin levels, sometimes used in galactagogue therapy under supervision.

Q99. Answer: B

Explanation: Mature milk contains roughly 60% whey and 40% casein, ensuring digestibility and balanced amino acid delivery. Colostrum starts with a higher whey proportion, gradually adjusting as lactation stabilizes.

Q100. Answer: B

Explanation: Auditory and tactile stimuli, especially infant crying and nipple touch, trigger oxytocin release via hypothalamic activation. This primes the let-down reflex even before feeding begins, ensuring efficient milk flow.

Questions (101-200)

Q101. Which maternal behavior most supports infant weight gain in the early postpartum period?
A. Offering both breasts per feeding
B. Scheduled feeding every 4 hours
C. Pumping once daily
D. Supplementing formula after each feed

Q102. Which feedback signal limits overproduction of milk in the mammary gland?
A. Oxytocin receptor downregulation
B. Feedback inhibitor of lactation (FIL)
C. Elevated dopamine release
D. Reduced blood prolactin

Q103. Which human milk mineral is most influenced by maternal dietary intake?
A. Calcium
B. Iron
C. Iodine
D. Zinc

Q104. Which maternal hormone promotes sodium reabsorption and may alter milk electrolyte balance postpartum?
A. Aldosterone
B. Cortisol
C. Estrogen
D. Prolactin

Q105. Which growth indicator most accurately reflects nutritional status in breastfed infants?
A. Head circumference
B. Length-for-age
C. Weight-for-length
D. Mid-upper arm circumference

Q106. Which hormone interacts with prolactin to promote alveolar differentiation and enzyme synthesis?
A. Insulin
B. Testosterone
C. Melatonin
D. Serotonin

Q107. Which maternal dietary deficiency leads to lower DHA content in breast milk?
A. Lack of seafood or omega-3 sources
B. Low iron intake
C. Excess carbohydrate intake
D. Vitamin C deficiency

Q108. Which factor is most essential for initiating lactogenesis II?
A. Estrogen surge
B. Drop in progesterone
C. Increase in oxytocin
D. Rise in cortisol

Q109. Which nutrient is most variable in human milk composition throughout a feeding?
A. Fat
B. Protein
C. Lactose

D. Sodium
Q110. Which gland secretes oxytocin into the bloodstream?
A. Anterior pituitary
B. Posterior pituitary
C. Hypothalamus directly
D. Pineal gland
Q111. Which maternal lifestyle factor most enhances vitamin D in milk?
A. Sunlight exposure
B. High-calcium diet
C. Sleep quality
D. Iron supplementation
Q112. Which hypothalamic-pituitary interaction regulates milk ejection reflexes?
A. Oxytocin inhibition loop
B. Neurohypophyseal activation
C. Adenohypophyseal suppression
D. Pineal-cortisol coordination
Q113. Which complementary feeding pattern minimizes anemia risk after six months?
A. Iron-rich purees with continued breastfeeding
B. Early cow's milk introduction
C. Exclusive breastfeeding until 12 months
D. Fruit-only feeding at weaning
Q114. Which hormone regulates maternal mood and stress tolerance during lactation?
A. Cortisol
B. Oxytocin
C. Adrenaline
D. Progesterone
Q115. Which feature of colostrum most benefits newborn immune protection?
A. High fat concentration
B. High immunoglobulin and leukocyte content
C. Low protein and mineral levels
D. Elevated lactose concentration
Q116. Which feedback mechanism terminates oxytocin release after feeding?
A. Sensory adaptation and neural cessation
B. Progesterone rise
C. Prolactin inhibition
D. Cortisol suppression
Q117. Which breast milk enzyme facilitates lipid digestion in infants?
A. Amylase
B. Lipase
C. Lactase
D. Protease
Q118. Which pituitary hormone modulates the stress response while indirectly supporting lactation?
A. ACTH
B. TSH
C. LH
D. FSH
Q119. Which human milk component is essential for infant intestinal epithelial repair?
A. Epidermal growth factor

B. Albumin
C. Lactose
D. Lysozyme

Q120. Which endocrine adaptation ensures sustained milk secretion during lactation maintenance?
A. Elevated baseline prolactin sensitivity
B. Rising progesterone concentration
C. Reduced oxytocin receptor activity
D. Increased dopamine inhibition

Q121. Which hormone primarily triggers milk ejection from the alveoli into the ducts during breastfeeding?
A. Estrogen
B. Prolactin
C. Oxytocin
D. Cortisol

Q122. Which pituitary hormone's secretion increases in response to nipple stimulation to sustain milk production?
A. FSH
B. LH
C. Prolactin
D. Oxytocin

Q123. In lactogenesis II, the onset of copious milk production is mainly triggered by which physiological change after birth?
A. Rise in estrogen
B. Drop in progesterone
C. Increase in cortisol
D. Decrease in prolactin

Q124. During lactation, dopamine acts as a:
A. Prolactin-stimulating hormone
B. Prolactin-inhibiting factor
C. Oxytocin agonist
D. Growth hormone substitute

Q125. Which maternal endocrine disorder is most commonly associated with delayed or insufficient milk production?
A. Addison's disease
B. Polycystic ovarian syndrome (PCOS)
C. Hypoglycemia
D. Graves' disease

Q126. Which hormone is essential for alveolar cell proliferation during pregnancy and early breast development?
A. Progesterone
B. Oxytocin
C. Dopamine
D. Insulin

Q127. Which mechanism best describes the milk ejection reflex?
A. Neural inhibition from hypothalamus to pituitary
B. Sensory input triggering posterior pituitary oxytocin release
C. Paracrine stimulation of alveolar growth
D. Chemical inhibition of prolactin

Q128. Which of the following hormones enhances lactose synthesis in mammary epithelial cells?
A. Prolactin
B. Oxytocin
C. Estrogen
D. Cortisol
Q129. Which maternal condition is most likely to cause hyperprolactinemia and galactorrhea outside of pregnancy?
A. Pituitary adenoma
B. Hypothyroidism
C. Cushing's syndrome
D. PCOS
Q130. Which hormone indirectly enhances prolactin's action by increasing mammary gland metabolic activity?
A. Cortisol
B. Dopamine
C. Testosterone
D. Melatonin
Q131. What is the physiological effect of sustained hyperprolactinemia postpartum?
A. Suppression of GnRH and fertility
B. Enhancement of ovarian follicle growth
C. Increased estrogen production
D. Activation of thyroid hormones
Q132. A mother with Sheehan's syndrome after postpartum hemorrhage is likely to have:
A. Elevated prolactin and normal lactation
B. Decreased prolactin and lactation failure
C. Increased TSH and hyperlactation
D. Normal oxytocin but poor milk ejection
Q133. Which maternal thyroid condition most commonly leads to low milk supply due to metabolic inefficiency?
A. Hyperthyroidism
B. Hypothyroidism
C. Thyroid carcinoma
D. Thyroiditis
Q134. In the context of lactation, which metabolic hormone works synergistically with prolactin to facilitate nutrient uptake by mammary cells?
A. Insulin
B. Adrenaline
C. Growth hormone
D. Thyroxine
Q135. What defines galactopoiesis in the lactation cycle?
A. Initiation of lactation post-delivery
B. Maintenance of ongoing milk secretion
C. Breast development during pregnancy
D. Withdrawal of progesterone inhibition
Q136. Which endocrine feedback primarily controls milk synthesis during established lactation?
A. Progesterone negative feedback
B. Autocrine control through local milk removal
C. Central hypothalamic inhibition

D. Estrogen receptor activation

Q137. Which mechanism explains how stress can inhibit milk ejection?

A. Decreased oxytocin secretion from the posterior pituitary
B. Increased dopamine blocking prolactin release
C. Decreased estrogen production
D. Suppressed alveolar growth

Q138. Which of the following is the most likely mechanism for lactation failure in pituitary necrosis?

A. Oxytocin receptor blockade
B. Prolactin deficiency
C. Estrogen excess
D. Dopamine hypersecretion

Q139. Which maternal factor most influences the onset of lactogenesis II after birth?

A. Frequency of early skin-to-skin contact
B. Maternal thyroid status
C. Uterine involution
D. Breast size before pregnancy

Q140. During lactation, which maternal hormone is most directly responsible for nutrient mobilization from body stores to support milk composition?

A. Cortisol
B. Glucagon
C. Insulin
D. Prolactin

Q141. Which infant condition most often results from poor latch leading to inadequate milk intake?

A. Gastroesophageal reflux
B. Hypoglycemia
C. Hyperbilirubinemia
D. Failure to thrive

Q142. What is the most likely cause of secondary lactation failure in a mother recovering from severe postpartum hemorrhage?

A. Adrenal overproduction
B. Pituitary ischemia
C. Thyroid hyperactivity
D. Mammary duct obstruction

Q143. Which infant pathology is directly linked with elevated unconjugated bilirubin and poor breastfeeding frequency?

A. Physiologic jaundice
B. Hemolytic anemia
C. Breastfeeding jaundice
D. Obstructive cholestasis

Q144. Which maternal breast condition is most often associated with fever, localized tenderness, and erythema?

A. Plugged duct
B. Mastitis
C. Galactocele
D. Engorgement

Q145. Which microbe most commonly causes infectious mastitis in lactating women?

A. Streptococcus pyogenes
B. Escherichia coli

C. Staphylococcus aureus
D. Candida albicans

Q146. What distinguishes a galactocele from an abscess during breast assessment?
A. Presence of milk fistula
B. Lack of inflammation and fluctuant fluid mass
C. Elevated temperature and pain
D. Pus drainage on aspiration

Q147. Which condition often results when a blocked duct remains untreated and infection develops?
A. Candidiasis
B. Mastitis
C. Fibrocystic changes
D. Ductal carcinoma

Q148. Which maternal symptom combination suggests breast abscess formation?
A. Breast firmness without redness
B. Painless lump and normal temperature
C. Fluctuant mass with fever after mastitis
D. Diffuse bilateral tenderness

Q149. In mastitis management, which is the best initial clinical action?
A. Stop breastfeeding immediately
B. Continue feeding and start antibiotics
C. Apply ice and bind breasts
D. Drain the breast surgically

Q150. Which antibiotic is most often prescribed for bacterial mastitis when MRSA is not suspected?
A. Vancomycin
B. Amoxicillin-clavulanate
C. Erythromycin
D. Ciprofloxacin

Q151. Which factor most contributes to nipple trauma during early breastfeeding?
A. Poor positioning
B. Excessive feeding duration
C. Overproduction of milk
D. Infant age over 3 months

Q152. Which underlying condition increases the risk of recurrent Candida nipple infection?
A. Maternal diabetes mellitus
B. Iron deficiency anemia
C. Postpartum hypertension
D. Hypothyroidism

Q153. Which sign differentiates Candida nipple infection from bacterial mastitis?
A. Diffuse swelling
B. Sharp, shooting breast pain after feeding
C. Fever and redness
D. Milk stasis and firmness

Q154. Which maternal condition most often leads to reduced milk volume and low supply despite normal latch?
A. Hypothyroidism
B. Engorgement
C. Overhydration
D. Nipple pain

Q155. What clinical feature differentiates plugged ducts from mastitis?
A. Fever and malaise
B. Localized tender lump without redness
C. Breast pain with lymphadenopathy
D. Discharge with foul odor
Q156. What is the most likely cause of persistent nipple pain after apparent healing of trauma?
A. Milk oversupply
B. Deep Candida infection
C. Ductal carcinoma
D. Recurrent mastitis
Q157. Which early symptom may indicate developing abscess during mastitis therapy?
A. Rapid fever resolution
B. Appearance of a fluctuant area
C. Decrease in milk output
D. Diffuse tenderness
Q158. In breastfeeding infants, which sign best indicates dehydration secondary to poor intake?
A. Soft fontanelle and decreased urination
B. Increased alertness
C. Frequent stools
D. Strong suck reflex
Q159. Which intervention prevents recurrence of plugged ducts in lactating women?
A. Limiting feeding frequency
B. Rotating feeding positions
C. Avoiding breast massage
D. Using tight bras
Q160. Which maternal factor is most likely to delay recovery from bacterial mastitis?
A. Early antibiotic initiation
B. Continued breastfeeding
C. Delayed milk drainage
D. Adequate rest and hydration
Q161. Which viral infection is an absolute contraindication to breastfeeding in developed settings due to transmission risk?
A. Hepatitis B
B. HIV
C. Cytomegalovirus (CMV)
D. Herpes simplex virus (HSV)
Q162. What is the safest feeding recommendation for an infant whose mother has active untreated tuberculosis?
A. Continue breastfeeding without precautions
B. Cease breastfeeding until mother is noninfectious
C. Formula feed permanently
D. Provide expressed milk during maternal isolation
Q163. Which maternal infection requires temporary cessation of breastfeeding due to potential toxicity of antiviral therapy?
A. Influenza
B. Herpes zoster (shingles) treated with valacyclovir
C. Cytomegalovirus
D. Meningitis treated with chloramphenicol

Q164. Which congenital infection can cause sensorineural hearing loss and jaundice in neonates?
A. Rubella
B. Toxoplasmosis
C. Cytomegalovirus (CMV)
D. Varicella
Q165. Which maternal metabolic condition is most likely to cause neonatal hypoglycemia during breastfeeding initiation?
A. Type 1 diabetes mellitus
B. Hypothyroidism
C. Cushing's syndrome
D. PCOS
Q166. Which breast abnormality presents as a firm, non-tender, fixed mass requiring biopsy to rule out malignancy?
A. Engorgement
B. Duct ectasia
C. Fibroadenoma
D. Carcinoma
Q167. Which bacterial pathogen is a common cause of late-onset neonatal sepsis in breastfeeding infants?
A. Group B Streptococcus
B. Listeria monocytogenes
C. Escherichia coli
D. Staphylococcus epidermidis
Q168. Which symptom triad is characteristic of infant hypocalcemia?
A. Lethargy, constipation, and cyanosis
B. Tremors, jitteriness, and seizures
C. Fever, irritability, and rash
D. Vomiting, diarrhea, and dehydration
Q169. Which maternal factor most predisposes to postpartum thyroiditis?
A. Multiparity
B. Type 1 diabetes
C. Obesity
D. Vitamin D deficiency
Q170. What is the most likely cause of delayed lactogenesis in a mother with retained placental fragments?
A. Excess estrogen
B. Persistent progesterone secretion
C. Elevated cortisol
D. Suppressed prolactin synthesis
Q171. Which condition in infants is often linked to maternal overproduction of milk and forceful let-down reflex?
A. Constipation
B. Colic and green frothy stools
C. Slow weight gain
D. Sleepiness and dehydration
Q172. Which finding suggests a congenital anomaly interfering with effective breastfeeding?
A. Tight lingual frenulum
B. Small mouth size

C. High-pitched cry
D. Mild nasal congestion

Q173. Which maternal autoimmune disorder often presents with recurrent low supply and fatigue?
A. Hashimoto's thyroiditis
B. Graves' disease
C. Lupus erythematosus
D. Rheumatoid arthritis

Q174. Which neonatal sign indicates possible cardiac pathology rather than feeding difficulty?
A. Poor latch
B. Cyanosis during feeding
C. Frequent spitting
D. Excessive crying

Q175. Which of the following may cause secondary lactation insufficiency despite normal hormonal function?
A. Retained placental tissue
B. Infrequent feeding
C. Hypopituitarism
D. Sheehan's syndrome

Q176. Which organism commonly causes thrush in breastfeeding dyads?
A. Staphylococcus aureus
B. Candida albicans
C. Group B Streptococcus
D. Pseudomonas aeruginosa

Q177. What finding is characteristic of infant gastroesophageal reflux rather than infection?
A. Projectile vomiting and fever
B. Effortless regurgitation with normal weight gain
C. Persistent diarrhea
D. Poor feeding and lethargy

Q178. Which factor most increases risk of neonatal jaundice during early breastfeeding?
A. Frequent feeds
B. Insufficient milk transfer
C. High maternal oxytocin
D. Early skin-to-skin contact

Q179. What best differentiates physiologic from pathologic jaundice in newborns?
A. Timing of onset
B. Skin color intensity
C. Presence of feeding difficulty
D. Response to sunlight exposure

Q180. Which condition involves inflammation of breast connective tissue extending beyond ducts and lobules?
A. Mastitis
B. Abscess
C. Cellulitis
D. Fibrocystic change

Q181. Which infant disorder is characterized by projectile non-bilious vomiting and palpable olive-shaped mass in the abdomen?
A. Gastroesophageal reflux
B. Pyloric stenosis

C. Intestinal obstruction
D. Hirschsprung disease
Q182. Which maternal condition increases risk for recurrent plugged ducts and mastitis?
A. Overhydration
B. Hyperlactation
C. Hypothyroidism
D. Mild dehydration
Q183. Which neonatal condition often presents with delayed meconium passage, abdominal distension, and bilious vomiting?
A. Hirschsprung disease
B. Gastroesophageal reflux
C. Intussusception
D. Meconium plug syndrome
Q184. A breastfeeding infant presents with lethargy and poor feeding after maternal antibiotic therapy. Which cause should be suspected?
A. Neonatal sepsis
B. Antibiotic transfer through milk causing gut flora alteration
C. Oral thrush
D. Cow's milk allergy
Q185. Which metabolic disorder presents with lethargy, poor feeding, and maple syrup odor in urine?
A. Phenylketonuria
B. Galactosemia
C. Maple syrup urine disease
D. Glycogen storage disease
Q186. What condition is most likely if a mother reports sharp breast pain and white nipple blanching after feeds?
A. Vasospasm (Raynaud's phenomenon)
B. Candidiasis
C. Mastitis
D. Plugged duct
Q187. Which maternal autoimmune disease may cause poor milk ejection due to antibody interference with oxytocin receptors?
A. Graves' disease
B. Lupus erythematosus
C. Multiple sclerosis
D. Rheumatoid arthritis
Q188. Which finding differentiates candidal nipple infection from Raynaud's vasospasm?
A. Color change of nipple
B. Pain triggered by cold
C. Deep burning pain post feeding
D. Relief with warmth
Q189. Which maternal condition leads to hyperlactation and frequent engorgement from excessive prolactin levels?
A. Pituitary adenoma
B. Hypothyroidism
C. Sheehan's syndrome
D. Type 1 diabetes
Q190. Which symptom pattern is typical of infant lactose overload syndrome?

A. Loose green frothy stools and gassiness
B. Hard pellet-like stools and straining
C. Vomiting and weight loss
D. Pale, clay-colored stools

Q191. Which breast condition is characterized by multiple tender nodules that wax and wane with hormonal changes?

A. Mastitis
B. Fibrocystic breast changes
C. Abscess
D. Duct ectasia

Q192. A breastfeeding mother with lupus nephritis is advised against which medication?

A. Prednisone
B. Hydroxychloroquine
C. Cyclophosphamide
D. Ibuprofen

Q193. Which infant sign indicates hypocalcemia related to maternal vitamin D deficiency?

A. High-pitched cry
B. Twitching and seizures
C. Persistent vomiting
D. Diarrhea

Q194. Which maternal factor increases risk of plugged ducts during lactation?

A. Wide-spaced nipples
B. Skipped feedings
C. Shallow areola
D. Increased hydration

Q195. Which condition may cause bilateral nipple discharge in a nonpregnant woman due to elevated prolactin?

A. Hypothyroidism
B. Pituitary adenoma
C. Cushing's syndrome
D. Diabetes mellitus

Q196. Which infant condition may require interruption of breastfeeding due to accumulation of toxic metabolites from galactose?

A. Maple syrup urine disease
B. Phenylketonuria
C. Galactosemia
D. Tyrosinemia

Q197. Which maternal breast condition shows nipple retraction and bloody discharge, raising concern for malignancy?

A. Duct ectasia
B. Intraductal papilloma
C. Fibroadenoma
D. Engorgement

Q198. Which lab finding supports diagnosis of postpartum thyroiditis in a lactating woman with fatigue and low milk supply?

A. Elevated TSH, low free T4
B. Decreased TSH, elevated T4
C. High prolactin, normal TSH

D. Low cortisol, normal T4

Q199. What is the safest antibiotic choice for treating mastitis during breastfeeding?

A. Trimethoprim-sulfamethoxazole

B. Amoxicillin-clavulanate

C. Doxycycline

D. Ciprofloxacin

Q200. Which maternal metabolic disorder can cause excessive fatigue and hypoglycemia during lactation?

A. Addison's disease

B. Cushing's syndrome

C. Hyperthyroidism

D. PCOS

Answer key and Explanation (101-200)

Q101. Answer: A

Explanation: Offering both breasts ensures full stimulation and balanced intake, maintaining prolactin response and milk volume. Scheduled or supplemental feeding may reduce supply through decreased natural demand.

Q102. Answer: B

Explanation: The Feedback Inhibitor of Lactation, a whey protein, accumulates in milk and suppresses further synthesis when alveoli are full. It provides local autocrine control, ensuring supply matches infant demand.

Q103. Answer: C

Explanation: Iodine content reflects maternal diet and supplementation more directly than calcium or iron, which remain stable. Insufficient iodine can impair infant thyroid and brain development.

Q104. Answer: A

Explanation: Aldosterone regulates sodium retention and indirectly affects milk composition during fluid shifts postpartum. Temporary electrolyte changes normalize as lactation stabilizes, maintaining consistent osmolarity.

Q105. Answer: C

Explanation: Weight-for-length assesses proportional growth and detects undernutrition or overnutrition. Head circumference and length progress more steadily, but weight changes reveal short-term energy balance.

Q106. Answer: A

Explanation: Insulin ensures adequate glucose uptake and lipid formation in mammary cells. It works with prolactin and cortisol to establish functional secretory capacity during lactogenesis I.

Q107. Answer: A

Explanation: Omega-3 fatty acids, particularly DHA, derive from marine and plant sources. Inadequate consumption lowers milk DHA, impacting infant neural and retinal development. Balanced maternal nutrition maintains optimal fatty acid profiles.

Q108. Answer: B

Explanation: Progesterone withdrawal after placental delivery removes inhibition on prolactin receptors, triggering onset of copious milk secretion. Oxytocin and cortisol support but do not initiate secretion.

Q109. Answer: A

Explanation: Fat concentration rises as the breast empties, delivering energy-dense hindmilk. Protein and lactose remain relatively stable. This natural gradient balances hydration and caloric supply.

Q110. Answer: B

Explanation: The posterior pituitary releases oxytocin synthesized in the hypothalamus. It travels via neural axons for systemic distribution, mediating milk ejection and maternal-infant bonding.

Q111. Answer: A

Explanation: Sunlight triggers dermal vitamin D synthesis, increasing maternal stores and milk concentration. Dietary intake alone rarely meets requirements, emphasizing outdoor exposure or supplementation for both mother and infant.

Q112. Answer: B

Explanation: Neurohypophyseal activation transmits neural stimuli from nipple mechanoreceptors to the posterior pituitary, prompting oxytocin release. This pathway ensures synchronized ejection from both breasts during feeding.

Q113. Answer: A

Explanation: Iron stores decline after six months; iron-fortified cereals or purees complement breast milk to prevent anemia. Cow's milk limits iron absorption and displaces breast milk prematurely.

Q114. Answer: B

Explanation: Oxytocin enhances relaxation, lowers stress hormone output, and fosters emotional bonding. This neurohormonal balance supports calm feeding interactions and postpartum mental well-being.

Q115. Answer: B

Explanation: Colostrum's immunoglobulin and leukocyte richness delivers passive immunity and intestinal protection. It coats mucosal surfaces, preventing infection during the newborn's early immunologically vulnerable period.

Q116. Answer: A

Explanation: When suckling stops, sensory input ceases, halting hypothalamic stimulation and oxytocin release. Hormonal feedback restores baseline levels, preventing unnecessary myoepithelial contractions.

Q117. Answer: B

Explanation: Human milk lipase breaks down triglycerides, compensating for immature pancreatic enzyme activity. This ensures efficient fat absorption and energy utilization essential for infant growth.

Q118. Answer: A

Explanation: ACTH stimulates cortisol secretion, which aids metabolic regulation during lactation. Moderate cortisol levels enhance lactogenesis, while chronic stress-induced excess may disrupt oxytocin reflexes.

Q119. Answer: A

Explanation: Epidermal growth factor (EGF) promotes mucosal regeneration and integrity, crucial for preventing enteric infections and necrotizing enterocolitis in preterm infants. Other proteins aid immunity but not epithelial renewal.

Q120. Answer: A

Explanation: Over time, prolactin receptors remain upregulated in alveolar cells, allowing sustained synthesis despite declining circulating hormone levels. This adaptation stabilizes production under normal feeding demand.

Q121. Answer: C

Explanation: Oxytocin causes contraction of myoepithelial cells surrounding alveoli, propelling milk into the ducts. Prolactin mainly regulates synthesis, not ejection. Estrogen and cortisol modulate gland development but don't initiate let-down. The oxytocin reflex depends on nipple stimulation and maternal emotional state.

Q122. Answer: C

Explanation: Prolactin is released from the anterior pituitary when the infant suckles, maintaining milk synthesis in alveolar cells. Oxytocin acts on ejection, not production. FSH and LH regulate ovarian function. Continuous nipple stimulation maintains prolactin levels and prevents suppression from dopamine.

Q123. Answer: B

Explanation: The drop in progesterone following placental delivery removes inhibition on prolactin receptors, allowing full activation of milk synthesis. Estrogen and cortisol support development but are not the key switch. Persistent high progesterone would delay milk coming in (delayed lactogenesis II).

Q124. Answer: B

Explanation: Dopamine from the hypothalamus inhibits prolactin release by acting on D2 receptors in the anterior pituitary. When suckling occurs, dopamine suppression allows prolactin surges. It's thus a prolactin-inhibiting factor, not a stimulant or oxytocin analog.

Q125. Answer: B

Explanation: PCOS can cause lactation insufficiency due to progesterone imbalance and insulin resistance disrupting mammary receptor signaling. Addison's affects cortisol balance; Graves' elevates thyroid hormones, rarely impairing milk directly. PCOS is most linked to poor milk supply outcomes.

Q126. Answer: A

Explanation: Progesterone, in concert with estrogen, drives lobuloalveolar proliferation during pregnancy, establishing lactation structures. Oxytocin triggers ejection; dopamine inhibits prolactin. Insulin supports metabolic readiness but not primary alveolar proliferation.

Q127. Answer: B

Explanation: Nipple stimulation activates sensory nerves sending impulses to the hypothalamus, causing the posterior pituitary to release oxytocin. This leads to myoepithelial contraction. It's a neuroendocrine reflex, not paracrine or inhibitory in nature.

Q128. Answer: A

Explanation: Prolactin upregulates lactose synthase enzyme expression, enabling lactose production and osmotic regulation of milk volume. Oxytocin mediates ejection, while estrogen and cortisol assist in structural development but don't directly control lactose synthesis.

Q129. Answer: A

Explanation: Prolactin-secreting pituitary adenomas (prolactinomas) produce excess prolactin independent of pregnancy, leading to galactorrhea. Hypothyroidism can mildly elevate prolactin due to TRH cross-stimulation, but adenoma is the primary pathological source.

Q130. Answer: A

Explanation: Cortisol synergizes with prolactin and insulin to optimize mammary metabolism, supporting protein and fat synthesis. Dopamine inhibits prolactin, testosterone has no lactogenic role, and melatonin's role in lactation remains minor and circadian.

Q131. Answer: A

Explanation: Elevated prolactin suppresses GnRH, reducing LH/FSH release, causing lactational amenorrhea. It's a natural contraceptive mechanism. Ovarian growth and estrogen production are decreased, not increased, during this period.

Q132. Answer: B

Explanation: Sheehan's syndrome causes anterior pituitary necrosis, reducing prolactin, leading to lactation failure. TSH and ACTH may also drop. Posterior pituitary oxytocin can remain intact, but without prolactin, milk synthesis ceases.

Q133. Answer: B

Explanation: Hypothyroidism decreases metabolic rate, reducing milk production efficiency and responsiveness to prolactin. Hyperthyroidism can cause irritability but doesn't impair synthesis directly. Replacement therapy usually restores supply.

Q134. Answer: A

Explanation: Insulin allows glucose and amino acid uptake into mammary epithelial cells, enabling prolactin-driven milk synthesis. Growth hormone indirectly supports metabolism, and thyroxine affects basal rate, not direct nutrient transfer.

Q135. Answer: B

Explanation: Galactopoiesis refers to the sustained secretion phase of milk production regulated mainly by prolactin and continual milk removal. Lactogenesis II is initiation, and mammogenesis is breast development.

Q136. Answer: B

Explanation: Established lactation depends on autocrine (local) control — the frequency and completeness of milk removal regulate synthesis. Systemic hormones play a secondary role once lactation stabilizes.

Q137. Answer: A

Explanation: Stress increases catecholamines that inhibit oxytocin release and its action on myoepithelial cells, disrupting let-down. Dopamine mainly affects prolactin, not ejection. Estrogen and alveolar changes are long-term factors.

Q138. Answer: B

Explanation: Pituitary necrosis destroys lactotrophs responsible for prolactin, halting milk production. Oxytocin release might continue, but without milk synthesis, ejection is irrelevant. Dopamine excess would also suppress but isn't the cause here.

Q139. Answer: A

Explanation: Early and frequent skin-to-skin contact promotes prolactin and oxytocin release, accelerating lactogenesis II. Thyroid and uterine changes are less directly related. Breast size doesn't predict functional milk production.

Q140. Answer: A

Explanation: Cortisol enhances lipolysis and gluconeogenesis, providing substrates for milk synthesis. Prolactin regulates synthesis within the breast but not systemic mobilization. Glucagon has minimal direct lactational impact.

Q141. Answer: D

Explanation: Inadequate latch reduces effective milk transfer, causing caloric deficiency and weight loss, leading to failure to thrive. Hyperbilirubinemia may follow but is secondary. Reflux and hypoglycemia are distinct metabolic conditions.

Q142. Answer: B

Explanation: Severe postpartum hemorrhage can cause pituitary ischemia (Sheehan's syndrome), damaging prolactin-secreting cells and halting milk production. Duct obstruction affects flow, not hormonal synthesis. Thyroid and adrenal changes are less relevant.

Q143. Answer: C

Explanation: Breastfeeding jaundice arises from infrequent feeding, reducing bilirubin excretion. It's a functional problem, not due to hemolysis or obstruction. Increasing feeds resolves it quickly, differentiating it from pathologic jaundice.

Q144. Answer: B

Explanation: Mastitis presents with inflammation, fever, and localized erythema, often from bacterial infection through nipple trauma. Plugged ducts lack systemic signs; engorgement is diffuse and noninfectious; galactocele is cystic without inflammation.

Q145. Answer: C

Explanation: Staphylococcus aureus is the leading pathogen in lactational mastitis due to colonization from infant oral flora. Candida causes thrush, not acute inflammation; E. coli and S. pyogenes are less frequent.

Q146. Answer: B

Explanation: A galactocele is a noninfectious milk-filled cyst without redness or fever. Abscesses contain pus, causing pain and systemic symptoms. Aspiration of galactocele yields sterile milk, confirming diagnosis.

Q147. Answer: B

Explanation: Stasis from an untreated blocked duct fosters bacterial growth, leading to mastitis. Fibrocystic and malignant conditions are unrelated. Candidiasis affects nipples but not ducts primarily.

Q148. Answer: C

Explanation: A fluctuant, tender mass with persistent fever after antibiotic therapy for mastitis suggests abscess. Aspiration confirms pus collection. Bilateral pain or firmness alone are not diagnostic.

Q149. Answer: B

Explanation: Continuing breastfeeding aids drainage and prevents stasis while antibiotics treat infection. Breast binding worsens retention; surgery is reserved for abscess. Early milk removal accelerates healing.

Q150. Answer: B

Explanation: Amoxicillin-clavulanate covers typical S. aureus and S. epidermidis pathogens. Vancomycin targets resistant strains; erythromycin is less effective for deep infection. Ciprofloxacin isn't preferred in lactation due to infant risk.

Q151. Answer: A
Explanation: Improper latch or positioning causes nipple friction, leading to fissures and infection risk. Duration alone doesn't cause trauma; overproduction causes engorgement. Correct technique prevents breakdown.
Q152. Answer: A
Explanation: Hyperglycemia in diabetes supports yeast growth, predisposing to Candida infections of nipple and ducts. Other conditions don't foster fungal proliferation directly. Glycemic control reduces recurrence.
Q153. Answer: B
Explanation: Candida causes deep, burning or shooting pain radiating after feeding, often with shiny or flaky nipple skin. Bacterial mastitis presents with redness, warmth, and systemic fever.
Q154. Answer: A
Explanation: Thyroid hormone deficiency decreases metabolic drive and prolactin receptor sensitivity, impairing milk synthesis. Engorgement and pain are mechanical; hydration rarely affects volume unless extreme.
Q155. Answer: B
Explanation: Plugged ducts present as localized, tender nodules without systemic symptoms or redness. Mastitis adds inflammation and fever. Infection-free massage and frequent feeding resolve plugs.
Q156. Answer: B
Explanation: Deep ductal Candida may persist even after superficial healing, causing sharp pain during and after feeding. Oversupply may cause fullness, not pain. Carcinoma rarely presents in early lactation.
Q157. Answer: B
Explanation: A newly palpable, fluctuant area during antibiotic treatment suggests abscess formation. Early detection allows drainage and continued lactation. Fever persistence and localized swelling confirm diagnosis.
Q158. Answer: A
Explanation: Dehydration manifests as sunken fontanelle, dry mucosa, and reduced wet diapers (<6/day). Frequent stools or alertness do not rule out fluid deficit. Monitoring output is key for early recognition.
Q159. Answer: B
Explanation: Rotating infant positions ensures complete milk drainage from all lobes, preventing duct blockage. Tight bras and infrequent feeds promote stasis. Gentle massage aids prevention.
Q160. Answer: C
Explanation: Delayed or incomplete drainage prolongs milk stasis, supporting bacterial growth and inflammation. Continued feeding with antibiotics accelerates recovery. Hydration supports healing but is secondary.
Q161. Answer: B
Explanation: HIV can be transmitted through breast milk; in areas with safe alternatives, breastfeeding is contraindicated. Hepatitis B and CMV are generally not contraindications with precautions. HSV requires covering active lesions only.
Q162. Answer: D
Explanation: Expressed milk remains safe since TB is not transmitted via milk, but close contact should be avoided until treatment renders the mother noninfectious. Once treated, direct feeding resumes safely.
Q163. Answer: D
Explanation: Chloramphenicol passes into milk and may cause gray baby syndrome, thus breastfeeding should pause during treatment. Valacyclovir and most antivirals are considered compatible; influenza transmission risk is low with precautions.
Q164. Answer: C

Explanation: Congenital CMV leads to hearing loss, jaundice, and hepatosplenomegaly. Rubella and toxoplasmosis cause different neurological manifestations. Varicella results in vesicular lesions, not jaundice.

Q165. Answer: A

Explanation: Infants of diabetic mothers are prone to hypoglycemia due to elevated fetal insulin after maternal hyperglycemia exposure. Early breastfeeding and glucose monitoring are essential preventive measures.

Q166. Answer: D

Explanation: A fixed, irregular, non-tender mass suggests carcinoma. Fibroadenoma is mobile and benign. Engorgement and duct ectasia are diffuse and soft. Any suspicious mass warrants biopsy.

Q167. Answer: A

Explanation: Group B Streptococcus often causes late-onset sepsis transmitted perinatally or postnatally. E. coli causes early sepsis; Listeria is rare. S. epidermidis typically causes mild infections in preterm infants.

Q168. Answer: B

Explanation: Neonatal hypocalcemia presents with tremors, jitteriness, and seizures due to low calcium affecting neuronal excitability. Other symptoms represent metabolic or infectious issues.

Q169. Answer: B

Explanation: Type 1 diabetes is an autoimmune disorder associated with higher incidence of postpartum thyroiditis due to immune cross-reactivity. Multiparity and vitamin D deficiency are not direct risk factors.

Q170. Answer: B

Explanation: Retained placental tissue continues to produce progesterone, inhibiting prolactin receptor activation and delaying milk onset. Removal normalizes endocrine feedback, restoring lactogenesis II.

Q171. Answer: B

Explanation: Overactive let-down causes infants to receive lactose-rich foremilk, resulting in gas, fussiness, and green stools. Management includes block feeding or expressing before feeding to moderate flow.

Q172. Answer: A

Explanation: Ankyloglossia (tongue-tie) restricts tongue movement, impairing latch and transfer efficiency. Mouth size and congestion may cause minor difficulty but not mechanical dysfunction.

Q173. Answer: A

Explanation: Hashimoto's thyroiditis leads to hypothyroidism, causing fatigue and low milk production. Graves' causes overactivity; lupus and rheumatoid arthritis primarily affect connective tissues, not lactation directly.

Q174. Answer: B

Explanation: Cyanosis with feeding suggests congenital heart disease affecting oxygenation. Poor latch or spitting may result from feeding mechanics, not cardiovascular compromise. Urgent evaluation is required.

Q175. Answer: B

Explanation: Infrequent milk removal suppresses supply due to autocrine feedback inhibition. Endocrine causes (Sheehan's, hypopituitarism) are primary failures. Frequent feeding reverses the suppression.

Q176. Answer: B

Explanation: Candida albicans infects nipples and infant mouths, causing pain and white plaques. S. aureus causes mastitis, not thrush. Group B Streptococcus and Pseudomonas rarely infect nipples.

Q177. Answer: B

Explanation: Physiologic reflux is common, with painless regurgitation and normal growth. Projectile vomiting or fever suggests pathology such as pyloric stenosis or infection.

Q178. Answer: B

Explanation: Insufficient intake delays meconium clearance and increases bilirubin reabsorption, leading to jaundice. Frequent feeding and early contact help prevent this condition.

Q179. Answer: A

Explanation: Physiologic jaundice appears after 24 hours of life and resolves spontaneously. Pathologic jaundice presents within the first day or persists longer than two weeks. Feeding issues may exacerbate both.

Q180. Answer: C

Explanation: Cellulitis affects the skin and subcutaneous tissues beyond glandular structures, presenting with diffuse redness and tenderness. Mastitis primarily involves ducts and lobules, while abscess forms a localized collection.

Q181. Answer: B

Explanation: Pyloric stenosis causes hypertrophy of the pylorus leading to obstruction, projectile vomiting, and visible peristalsis. Reflux lacks projectile force; obstruction shows bilious emesis. Palpable mass confirms diagnosis.

Q182. Answer: B

Explanation: Hyperlactation creates milk stasis and engorgement, predisposing to duct blockage and infection. Hypothyroidism reduces supply, while hydration levels are secondary influences.

Q183. Answer: A

Explanation: Hirschsprung disease results from absence of enteric ganglion cells, preventing stool passage and causing distension. Intussusception presents later with currant-jelly stools. Early diagnosis requires surgical evaluation.

Q184. Answer: B

Explanation: Certain antibiotics alter gut microbiota when transferred via milk, leading to GI upset and lethargy. Sepsis presents with systemic signs. Thrush or allergies show different local symptoms.

Q185. Answer: C

Explanation: Maple syrup urine disease involves defective branched-chain amino acid metabolism, producing characteristic odor and CNS depression. Early detection prevents neurological damage. Breastfeeding may continue if diet adjusted.

Q186. Answer: A

Explanation: Vasospasm causes nipple blanching, color change, and sharp pain triggered by cold or trauma. Candida causes deep burning pain without blanching. Mastitis adds systemic fever and erythema.

Q187. Answer: C

Explanation: In multiple sclerosis, autoimmune disruption of neural transmission and oxytocin receptor sensitivity can impair let-down reflex. Lupus and rheumatoid arthritis mainly affect systemic tissues, not oxytocin function.

Q188. Answer: C

Explanation: Candida infection causes persistent deep pain after feeding regardless of temperature. Vasospasm pain is cold-sensitive and improves with warmth. Color change indicates vascular involvement.

Q189. Answer: A

Explanation: Prolactinomas overproduce prolactin, causing galactorrhea and engorgement. Sheehan's and hypothyroidism cause low supply. Diabetes affects glucose regulation, not direct prolactin output.

Q190. Answer: A

Explanation: Excess foremilk intake from rapid let-down leads to high lactose exposure causing gas and frothy stools. Clay stools suggest liver disease; hard stools indicate constipation.

Q191. Answer: B

Explanation: Fibrocystic changes are benign nodularities fluctuating with the menstrual cycle. They're tender but noninfectious. Mastitis and abscess have acute inflammation, while duct ectasia causes sticky discharge.

Q192. Answer: C

Explanation: Cyclophosphamide is cytotoxic and contraindicated during lactation due to risk of bone marrow suppression in infants. Prednisone and hydroxychloroquine are generally safe at standard doses.

Q193. Answer: B
Explanation: Neonatal hypocalcemia manifests with neuromuscular irritability—tremors, twitching, and seizures. Vitamin D deficiency impairs calcium absorption. Crying or vomiting may accompany but aren't diagnostic.
Q194. Answer: B
Explanation: Skipping feeds promotes milk stasis leading to duct blockage. Regular and complete drainage prevents recurrence. Anatomic variations alone seldom cause obstruction.
Q195. Answer: B
Explanation: Pituitary prolactinomas secrete prolactin independent of pregnancy, causing galactorrhea. Hypothyroidism may elevate prolactin mildly via TRH stimulation but less severely.
Q196. Answer: C
Explanation: Classic galactosemia results from GALT deficiency, preventing galactose metabolism. Lactose-containing milk becomes toxic; soy formula is required. PKU and tyrosinemia allow breastfeeding with monitoring.
Q197. Answer: B
Explanation: Intraductal papilloma presents with unilateral bloody nipple discharge without mass. Duct ectasia causes sticky non-bloody discharge; fibroadenoma and engorgement lack discharge.
Q198. Answer: A
Explanation: Autoimmune thyroiditis leads to hypothyroid phase marked by high TSH and low free T4. Fatigue and low milk output follow metabolic slowdown. Correction improves lactation.
Q199. Answer: B
Explanation: Amoxicillin-clavulanate covers staphylococcal infections and is safe for infants. Doxycycline and fluoroquinolones are avoided due to bone and cartilage toxicity risks. TMP-SMX used only if no neonatal jaundice.
Q200. Answer: A
Explanation: Addison's disease (adrenal insufficiency) results in cortisol deficiency, causing fatigue and hypoglycemia. It can impair lactation through low metabolic support. Replacement therapy restores balance.

Questions (201-300)

Q201. A breastfeeding mother develops mastitis with localized redness and fever. What is the most appropriate initial management?

A. Begin corticosteroid therapy
B. Stop all feeds and switch to formula
C. Apply ice and avoid touching the breast
D. Continue breastfeeding and initiate antibiotics if symptoms persist 24–48 hours

Q202. Which infant condition most interferes with milk transfer?

A. Ankyloglossia (tongue-tie)
B. Mild nasal congestion
C. Cradle cap
D. Diaper rash

Q203. A mother presents with nipple pain and shiny, flaky skin. Infant shows white oral patches. Likely cause is:

A. Candidal infection
B. Eczema
C. Milk bleb
D. Poor hygiene

Q204. Which symptom distinguishes plugged duct from mastitis?

A. Absence of systemic fever
B. Red streaks on breast
C. Generalized malaise
D. Nipple discharge with odor

Q205. A mother with diabetes develops delayed lactogenesis II. Primary contributing factor is:

A. Excessive caffeine intake
B. Low hydration status
C. Poor diet quality
D. Hormonal imbalance affecting insulin and prolactin interaction

Q206. Which maternal condition is a contraindication to breastfeeding?

A. HIV infection in resource-rich settings
B. Controlled hypothyroidism
C. Mastitis under antibiotic therapy
D. Hepatitis B infection

Q207. An infant presents with yellowing skin and sclera on day three. What should be assessed first?

A. Feeding frequency and latch effectiveness
B. Infant bowel pattern only
C. Maternal hydration
D. Skin care products used

Q208. Which breast condition requires immediate drainage to prevent complications?

A. Abscess
B. Engorgement
C. Milk blister
D. Fibroadenoma

Q209. A preterm infant exhibits hypoglycemia. The IBCLC's immediate role is to:

A. Use glucose water as substitute
B. Delay feeding until glucose stabilizes
C. Recommend IV fluids only

D. Encourage early and frequent feeding or expressed colostrum

Q210. Nipple blanching and pain after feeding suggest:

A. Vasospasm (Raynaud's phenomenon)
B. Candida infection
C. Eczema
D. Ductal obstruction

Q211. Which infant symptom indicates potential cardiac anomaly affecting feeding?

A. Fatigue and diaphoresis during feeding
B. Crying after burping
C. Occasional hiccups
D. Preference for one breast

Q212. Which maternal breast anomaly can reduce effective milk removal?

A. Hypoplastic (insufficient glandular) tissue
B. Symmetrical enlargement
C. Nipple pigmentation
D. Stretch marks

Q213. A newborn with cleft palate struggles to maintain suction. Appropriate feeding intervention is:

A. Using rigid nipple shields
B. Attempting exclusive direct breastfeeding
C. Specialized feeder or upright positioning with pacing
D. Forcing latch repeatedly

Q214. What condition most often mimics mastitis but results from milk stasis alone?

A. Engorgement
B. Breast abscess
C. Fungal infection
D. Cellulitis

Q215. Which endocrine disorder most interferes with lactation?

A. Polycystic ovarian syndrome (PCOS)
B. Hyperlipidemia
C. Anemia
D. Vitamin D deficiency

Q216. An infant diagnosed with GERD exhibits back arching and crying at breast. Management includes:

A. Upright feeding and smaller, frequent feeds
B. Restricting feeding volume drastically
C. Using thickened formula instead of breastmilk
D. Continuous supine feeding

Q217. A mother reports recurring plugged ducts on the same side. What should be evaluated?

A. Maternal diet variety
B. Maternal hydration alone
C. Baby's birth weight
D. Bra pressure or infant position consistency

Q218. What infant factor increases risk of dehydration in the first week?

A. Ineffective latch and infrequent feeding
B. High environmental humidity
C. Maternal diet composition
D. Rapid weight gain

Q219. Which medication class most commonly suppresses lactation?

A. Estrogen-containing contraceptives

B. Thyroid replacement hormones
C. Nonsteroidal anti-inflammatories
D. Iron supplements

Q220. A mother recovering from cesarean section develops delayed initiation of breastfeeding. Key supportive strategy is:
A. Encourage skin-to-skin and assist comfortable positioning despite incision pain
B. Delay feeds until pain subsides fully
C. Restrict feeding to one breast
D. Avoid movement for several days

Q221. Which medication used for migraines is contraindicated during lactation due to risk of infant apnea?
A. Sumatriptan
B. Ergotamine
C. Acetaminophen
D. Ibuprofen

Q222. Which maternal behavior increases lead exposure risk through breast milk?
A. Use of ceramic cookware with old glaze
B. Frequent exercise
C. Vegetarian diet
D. High calcium intake

Q223. Which maternal substance can accumulate in breast milk and cause infant sedation and hypotonia?
A. Alcohol
B. Cannabis
C. Nicotine
D. Caffeine

Q224. Which antibiotic is considered the drug of choice for postpartum endometritis during breastfeeding?
A. Clindamycin
B. Doxycycline
C. Ciprofloxacin
D. Chloramphenicol

Q225. What is the safest strategy to minimize infant exposure when a mother must take a potentially risky medication?
A. Increase maternal dose
B. Stop feeding permanently
C. Time breastfeeding immediately before dosing
D. Pump and store milk after dosing

Q226. Which maternal exposure can cause cyanosis and methemoglobinemia in infants via breast milk?
A. Nitrate-contaminated water
B. Excess iron
C. Vitamin D supplements
D. Herbal teas

Q227. Which type of radiologic contrast requires no interruption of breastfeeding?
A. Iodine-131
B. Gadolinium MRI contrast
C. Technetium-99m
D. Thallium scan

Q228. Which maternal habit is most associated with decreased milk production due to vasoconstriction of mammary vessels?
A. Alcohol use
B. Smoking
C. Excess caffeine
D. Vegan diet
Q229. Which commonly used over-the-counter medication may suppress lactation due to anticholinergic properties?
A. Loratadine
B. Pseudoephedrine
C. Ranitidine
D. Diphenhydramine
Q230. Which herbal galactagogue may cause hypoglycemia and allergic reactions in some users?
A. Fenugreek
B. Blessed thistle
C. Goat's rue
D. Fennel
Q231. Which type of maternal diet most risks deficiency in DHA and vitamin B12 affecting infant neurodevelopment?
A. Vegan diet without supplementation
B. Gluten-free diet
C. Low-fat diet
D. High-protein diet
Q232. Which class of antihypertensive drugs should be avoided during lactation due to risk of infant bradycardia?
A. Beta-blockers (e.g., atenolol)
B. Calcium channel blockers
C. ACE inhibitors
D. Diuretics
Q233. Which maternal toxin causes neurodevelopmental delay and accumulates in fatty tissues, concentrating in breast milk?
A. Lead
B. Mercury
C. Arsenic
D. Cadmium
Q234. Which maternal medication should be withheld 12–24 hours before breastfeeding resumes after radioactive testing?
A. Technetium-99m
B. Iodine-131
C. Thallium
D. Gadolinium
Q235. Which infant effect can occur with excessive maternal caffeine intake (>300 mg/day)?
A. Sleep disturbance and irritability
B. Hypoglycemia
C. Sedation
D. Bradycardia
Q236. Which topical medication is unsafe during lactation due to risk of infant methemoglobinemia if ingested?

A. Lidocaine
B. Benzocaine
C. Hydrocortisone
D. Lanolin

Q237. Which antibiotic is contraindicated in infants under two months due to risk of kernicterus?
A. Erythromycin
B. Trimethoprim-sulfamethoxazole
C. Cephalexin
D. Penicillin

Q238. Which drug is recommended to treat postpartum depression in lactating women with minimal infant sedation?
A. Sertraline
B. Paroxetine
C. Nortriptyline
D. Fluoxetine

Q239. Which environmental contaminant can accumulate in breast milk fat and affect infant endocrine function?
A. Dioxins
B. Nitrates
C. Asbestos
D. Iron

Q240. Which pharmacologic principle most influences drug transfer into breast milk?
A. Protein binding and lipid solubility
B. Molecular weight alone
C. Route of administration
D. Duration of treatment

Q241. A breastfeeding mother presents with fever, breast tenderness, and localized erythema. What is the first-line management for mastitis?
A. Stop breastfeeding immediately
B. Begin warm compresses only
C. Continue breastfeeding and start appropriate antibiotics
D. Use tight binding to suppress lactation

Q242. Which factor most commonly predisposes to recurrent plugged ducts?
A. Maternal obesity
B. Skipped feedings and poor drainage
C. Elevated prolactin
D. Overhydration

Q243. A firm, fluctuant mass develops following untreated mastitis. What is the diagnosis?
A. Galactocele
B. Abscess
C. Fibroadenoma
D. Plugged duct

Q244. Nipple thrush should be suspected when the mother reports:
A. Sharp, burning nipple pain persisting between feeds
B. Mild tenderness with engorgement
C. Red streaks radiating from the nipple
D. Local warmth and purulent drainage

Q245. Which statement best describes management of breast abscess?

A. Stop nursing completely
B. Drain abscess and continue breastfeeding if possible
C. Suppress lactation with dopamine agonists
D. Apply ice and pressure only

Q246. What finding differentiates milk bleb from mastitis?
A. Systemic symptoms
B. Pus discharge
C. Small white blister on nipple surface
D. Breast erythema

Q247. Which maternal condition contraindicates breastfeeding?
A. Mastitis
B. Hepatitis B with infant prophylaxis
C. HIV infection where safe alternatives exist
D. Herpes on the leg

Q248. A 2-week-old infant has persistent jaundice but is thriving and feeding well. Diagnosis?
A. Pathologic jaundice
B. Breast milk jaundice
C. Hemolytic anemia
D. Infection

Q249. Early-onset breastfeeding jaundice is usually related to:
A. Breast milk composition
B. Poor milk intake and dehydration
C. Genetic polymorphisms
D. Hepatic disease

Q250. A postpartum woman with nipple trauma develops severe pain and erythema extending outward in streaks. What is most likely?
A. Dermatitis
B. Vasospasm
C. Candidiasis
D. Bacterial mastitis

Q251. Fibrocystic breast changes are characterized by:
A. Hard, immobile lump
B. Fluctuating cystic nodules tender before menses
C. Warmth and redness
D. Nipple discharge only

Q252. A neonate with yellow-green emesis and poor feeding after birth should be assessed for:
A. GERD
B. Intestinal obstruction
C. Physiologic reflux
D. Milk oversupply

Q253. Which finding suggests ankyloglossia affecting breastfeeding?
A. Shallow latch and maternal nipple pain
B. Rapid infant weight gain
C. Excessive spit-up
D. Constant crying after feeding

Q254. Maternal diabetes is associated with increased risk of:
A. Neonatal hypoglycemia
B. Delayed cord separation

C. Polycythemia only
D. Rapid lactogenesis II

Q255. A mother reports burning nipple pain that worsens in cold weather with blanching. Likely cause?
A. Vasospasm (Raynaud phenomenon)
B. Candidiasis
C. Eczema
D. Plugged duct

Q256. Which infant condition may require temporary breastfeeding interruption?
A. Cytomegalovirus in full-term infants
B. Herpes simplex lesion on mother's breast
C. Maternal cold
D. Mild jaundice

Q257. The best indicator of adequate breastfeeding in an infant with slow weight gain is:
A. Number of feeds
B. Audible swallowing and output
C. Maternal breast fullness
D. Infant sleep duration

Q258. A galactocele differs from an abscess in that:
A. It contains milk, not pus
B. It is red and painful
C. It requires antibiotics
D. It causes systemic symptoms

Q259. Which maternal autoimmune disease may reduce milk supply?
A. Graves disease
B. Lupus erythematosus
C. Hashimoto thyroiditis
D. Rheumatoid arthritis

Q260. What is the most appropriate management for nipple eczema?
A. Topical steroids compatible with breastfeeding
B. Discontinue breastfeeding
C. Oral antifungal medication
D. Antihistamines only

Q261. What is the primary management goal in subclinical mastitis?
A. Improve milk flow and reduce inflammation
B. Stop breastfeeding immediately
C. Apply tight compression
D. Use prophylactic antibiotics continuously

Q262. A mother presents with cracked nipples and Candida infection. The best intervention includes:
A. Treating both mother and infant with antifungal therapy
B. Discontinuing breastfeeding
C. Applying topical steroids only
D. Increasing pump suction

Q263. What differentiates bacterial mastitis from blocked ducts?
A. Absence of erythema
B. Localized lump only
C. Systemic symptoms such as fever and malaise
D. No discomfort

Q264. Which condition commonly mimics inflammatory breast cancer during lactation?

A. Severe infectious mastitis
B. Galactocele
C. Subareolar abscess
D. Fibroadenoma

Q265. What is the safest analgesic for breastfeeding mothers with mastitis?
A. Ibuprofen
B. Aspirin
C. Codeine
D. Oxycodone

Q266. What is a key preventive strategy for recurrent mastitis?
A. Correct latch and avoid tight clothing
B. Reduce feeding frequency
C. Wean early
D. Use antibiotics prophylactically

Q267. Which maternal factor delays lactogenesis II?
A. Immediate postpartum feeding
B. Frequent skin-to-skin contact
C. Retained placental fragments
D. Maternal hydration

Q268. When evaluating greenish breast milk, what is the likely cause?
A. Benign dietary pigment from leafy vegetables
B. Bacterial infection
C. Blood contamination
D. Medication reaction

Q269. Which drug is contraindicated during lactation due to infant sedation risk?
A. Codeine
B. Acetaminophen
C. Ibuprofen
D. Dicloxacillin

Q270. When prescribing antibiotics for mastitis, the IBCLC should confirm:
A. Compatibility with breastfeeding
B. Stopping milk expression
C. Use of broad-spectrum agents only
D. Extended high-dose regimens

Q271. What defines a galactocele?
A. Hormonal tumor
B. Infectious abscess
C. Fibrotic lesion
D. Milk-filled cyst due to ductal blockage

Q272. Which maternal endocrine disorder most commonly lowers milk supply?
A. Hypothyroidism
B. Diabetes mellitus
C. Hyperprolactinemia
D. Addison's disease

Q273. Which medication supports prolactin secretion in induced lactation protocols?
A. Domperidone
B. Pseudoephedrine
C. Bromocriptine

D. Decongestants

Q274. What is the primary symptom of Raynaud's phenomenon of the nipple?

A. Sharp, burning pain with color change
B. Constant dull ache
C. Itching without blanching
D. Swelling of areola only

Q275. Which over-the-counter medication can reduce milk supply?

A. Docusate sodium
B. Ibuprofen
C. Loratadine
D. Pseudoephedrine

Q276. Which herbal galactagogue has the strongest clinical support for modest milk increase?

A. Fenugreek
B. Black cohosh
C. Ginkgo biloba
D. St. John's wort

Q277. Which maternal condition requires close monitoring when using domperidone?

A. Cardiac arrhythmia
B. Mild dehydration
C. Low body weight
D. Iron deficiency

Q278. Which environmental toxin can accumulate in breast milk and pose risk to infants?

A. Polychlorinated biphenyls (PCBs)
B. Sodium chloride
C. Calcium carbonate
D. Plant starches

Q279. Which property increases drug transfer into breast milk?

A. High protein binding
B. High lipid solubility
C. High molecular weight
D. Low pKa

Q280. What is the safest analgesic for breastfeeding mothers?

A. Codeine
B. Ibuprofen
C. Oxycodone
D. Aspirin

Q281. Which antibiotic is generally considered safe during lactation?

A. Tetracycline
B. Ciprofloxacin
C. Amoxicillin
D. Chloramphenicol

Q282. Which antidepressant has the most safety data in breastfeeding?

A. Paroxetine
B. Fluoxetine
C. Sertraline
D. Citalopram

Q283. Which contraceptive option is preferred for breastfeeding women under 6 months postpartum?

A. Combined estrogen–progestin pill

B. Progestin-only method
C. Copper IUD contraindicated
D. Vaginal ring

Q284. Galactagogues act primarily by increasing:
A. Progesterone
B. Prolactin secretion
C. Estrogen levels
D. Dopamine

Q285. Herbal galactagogues with limited evidence include:
A. Fenugreek and milk thistle
B. Valerian and ginger
C. Chamomile and peppermint
D. St. John's wort and ginseng

Q286. Which substance is most likely to reduce milk supply?
A. Domperidone
B. Pseudoephedrine
C. Metoclopramide
D. Fenugreek

Q287. What is the recommendation for breastfeeding after maternal alcohol consumption?
A. Stop breastfeeding for 24 hours
B. Resume feeding once clinically sober
C. Pump and dump for two days
D. Give formula for one feeding only

Q288. Nicotine exposure through breastfeeding may cause:
A. Improved sleep
B. Increased heart rate and restlessness
C. Hypothermia
D. Constipation

Q289. Which statement regarding cannabis and breastfeeding is accurate?
A. THC does not enter breast milk
B. THC is fat-soluble and accumulates in milk
C. CBD neutralizes THC risk
D. Short-term exposure is harmless

Q290. Which radioactive procedure requires temporary cessation of breastfeeding?
A. Chest X-ray
B. MRI without contrast
C. Iodine-131 therapy
D. Ultrasound

Q291. Which drug is contraindicated during breastfeeding due to risk of infant aplastic anemia?
A. Amoxicillin
B. Chloramphenicol
C. Metronidazole
D. Cefalexin

Q292. What effect do dopamine agonists like bromocriptine have on lactation?
A. Stimulate milk production
B. Suppress prolactin and inhibit lactation
C. Increase oxytocin
D. Reduce breast pain only

Q293. Which anticonvulsant requires caution due to sedation and poor feeding in infants?
A. Valproate
B. Lamotrigine
C. Carbamazepine
D. Phenobarbital
Q294. The milk-to-plasma ratio indicates:
A. Maternal drug tolerance
B. Extent of drug transfer to milk
C. Infant hepatic clearance
D. Breast storage time
Q295. Which antipsychotic is least likely to cause infant sedation?
A. Haloperidol
B. Clozapine
C. Risperidone
D. Olanzapine
Q296. When advising a lactating woman prescribed a new medication, the consultant should:
A. Automatically advise cessation of breastfeeding
B. Consult evidence-based lactation pharmacology resources
C. Rely on package insert warnings only
D. Suggest formula supplementation
Q297. Which herbal supplement may decrease milk supply?
A. Sage
B. Fenugreek
C. Blessed thistle
D. Alfalfa
Q298. What is the safest antihypertensive for a breastfeeding mother?
A. Lisinopril
B. Methyldopa
C. Enalapril
D. Atenolol
Q299. Which analgesic is contraindicated due to infant risk of Reye's syndrome?
A. Acetaminophen
B. Ibuprofen
C. Aspirin
D. Naproxen
Q300. What should be done when a breastfeeding mother is prescribed chemotherapy?
A. Continue feeding normally
B. Pump and store milk during therapy
C. Stop breastfeeding during and after treatment
D. Feed immediately post-infusion

Answer key and Explanation (201-300)

Q201. Answer: D

Explanation: Continued breastfeeding aids drainage and prevents abscess formation. Antibiotics follow persistent infection. Cessation worsens engorgement and inflammation. Ice may soothe, but stopping feeds increases pressure and bacterial load.

Q202. Answer: A

Explanation: Restricted tongue mobility hinders latch depth and suction efficiency. Nasal congestion can cause temporary disruption, but tongue-tie directly limits feeding mechanics. Skin or diaper issues are unrelated to oral transfer function.

Q203. Answer: A

Explanation: Fungal infection produces burning pain, shiny tissue, and thrush in infant's mouth. Eczema lacks oral lesions; blebs are localized. Hygiene alone does not cause candidiasis, which thrives in warm, moist conditions.

Q204. Answer: A

Explanation: Plugged ducts cause localized tenderness without systemic signs. Mastitis presents with fever and inflammation spread. Odor and discharge suggest infection or abscess rather than mechanical obstruction.

Q205. Answer: D

Explanation: Insulin resistance disrupts prolactin and cortisol coordination essential for milk onset. Hydration and diet play minor roles. Managing glucose levels and initiating frequent feeding stimulate hormonal normalization.

Q206. Answer: A

Explanation: HIV transmission risk warrants avoidance where safe alternatives exist. Treated thyroid conditions and hepatitis B are not absolute contraindications. Mastitis with antibiotics allows continued feeding.

Q207. Answer: A

Explanation: Early jaundice often results from poor intake and dehydration. Effective feeding promotes bilirubin excretion through stool. Skin products rarely influence jaundice; hydration alone is insufficient without milk transfer improvement.

Q208. Answer: A

Explanation: Abscesses form from untreated mastitis, demanding surgical or needle drainage to relieve pain and restore function. Engorgement and blisters resolve conservatively. Fibroadenomas are benign and noninfectious.

Q209. Answer: D

Explanation: Early colostrum intake stabilizes blood sugar and supports gut development. Delays or substitutes lack nutrient density and immune factors. Collaboration with medical team ensures metabolic stability and feeding coordination.

Q210. Answer: A

Explanation: Vasospasm causes sharp pain and color changes triggered by cold or compression. Candida lacks blanching; eczema appears as itching. Managing warmth and reducing nipple trauma alleviates symptoms effectively.

Q211. Answer: A

Explanation: Diaphoresis and poor endurance reflect circulatory stress during feeding, a classic cardiac sign. Other responses are normal variations. Immediate referral ensures diagnostic evaluation and safety.

Q212. Answer: A

Explanation: Limited glandular development restricts storage and synthesis capacity. Pigmentation and stretch marks are cosmetic. Identifying true hypoplasia allows targeted management and realistic expectation setting.

Q213. Answer: C
Explanation: Specialized feeders and upright pacing compensate for structural gaps and aspiration risk. Forced direct feeding can cause distress. Adaptive technique ensures nutrition while preserving mother-infant bonding.
Q214. Answer: A
Explanation: Engorgement causes firm, tender breasts without infection. Distinguishing from mastitis avoids unnecessary antibiotics. Abscesses and cellulitis present with systemic illness or purulent discharge.
Q215. Answer: A
Explanation: PCOS disrupts progesterone and prolactin balance essential for milk synthesis. Nutrient deficiencies and metabolic disorders affect health indirectly but seldom suppress lactogenesis significantly.
Q216. Answer: A
Explanation: Upright feeding reduces reflux and discomfort. Breastmilk digestion is faster than formula, lessening irritation. Supine feeding increases regurgitation risk; drastic volume restriction causes inadequate intake.
Q217. Answer: D
Explanation: External compression or repetitive positioning restricts ductal drainage. Identifying physical contributors prevents chronic obstruction. Hydration or diet rarely cause localized, repeated blockage patterns.
Q218. Answer: A
Explanation: Poor intake leads to reduced urine output and jaundice. Environmental or maternal diet factors are minimal contributors. Frequent effective feeding maintains hydration and metabolism.
Q219. Answer: A
Explanation: Estrogens antagonize prolactin, reducing milk production. Thyroid or iron therapies maintain general health and do not directly inhibit lactation. NSAIDs manage pain safely during breastfeeding.
Q220. Answer: A
Explanation: Early contact and adaptive positioning overcome surgical limitations and stimulate hormonal lactogenesis. Delay prolongs milk onset. Comfort-focused assistance promotes success and recovery.
Q221. Answer: B
Explanation: Ergotamine suppresses prolactin and may cause infant apnea and vomiting. Sumatriptan has low milk transfer and is considered compatible. Acetaminophen and ibuprofen are safe analgesics.
Q222. Answer: A
Explanation: Lead leaches from improperly glazed ceramics and accumulates in bone, mobilizing during lactation. Exercise or diet are less significant factors. Calcium intake reduces lead absorption.
Q223. Answer: B
Explanation: THC from cannabis concentrates in breast milk, leading to infant sedation and reduced motor tone. Alcohol effects are transient; nicotine stimulates, and caffeine causes irritability, not sedation.
Q224. Answer: A
Explanation: Clindamycin effectively covers anaerobes and Gram-positive organisms and is compatible with lactation. Doxycycline and chloramphenicol are avoided for infant bone marrow or tooth effects.
Q225. Answer: C
Explanation: Feeding before dosing allows drug metabolism before next feed, minimizing infant exposure. Pumping post-dose may increase exposure. Permanent cessation is unnecessary for short-term therapy.
Q226. Answer: A
Explanation: Nitrates convert hemoglobin to methemoglobin, impairing oxygen transport. Infants are highly sensitive. Proper water filtration prevents toxicity. Other listed exposures are safe in moderation.
Q227. Answer: B
Explanation: Gadolinium-based contrast is minimally absorbed orally by infants. Radioisotopes like iodine and technetium require temporary cessation. MRI contrast allows immediate feeding post-scan.

Q228. Answer: B
Explanation: Nicotine-induced vasoconstriction reduces mammary blood flow and prolactin levels, impairing supply. Alcohol affects ejection transiently; caffeine and diet have lesser effects.
Q229. Answer: B
Explanation: Pseudoephedrine reduces milk supply through vasoconstriction and dopamine-mediated prolactin inhibition. Loratadine and ranitidine are safe alternatives; diphenhydramine causes infant sedation but less supply impact.
Q230. Answer: A
Explanation: Fenugreek may lower blood sugar and trigger allergic symptoms, especially in individuals sensitive to legumes. Evidence for milk enhancement remains inconclusive.
Q231. Answer: A
Explanation: Vegan diets lack DHA and B12 sources unless fortified, risking infant developmental delays. Balanced plant-based diets with supplements remain compatible with lactation.
Q232. Answer: A
Explanation: Beta-blockers like atenolol transfer into milk and can cause bradycardia and lethargy in infants. Nifedipine and ACE inhibitors are generally safer options postnatally.
Q233. Answer: B
Explanation: Methylmercury from fish concentrates in fat-rich milk, leading to potential neurotoxicity. Lead and cadmium also pose risks but are less lipophilic. Dietary caution prevents exposure.
Q234. Answer: A
Explanation: Technetium-99m requires short-term milk discard (12–24 hours) to prevent infant exposure. Iodine-131 requires longer cessation; gadolinium is safe for immediate feeding.
Q235. Answer: A
Explanation: High caffeine intake leads to irritability and insomnia in infants due to immature metabolism. Moderate intake (<200 mg/day) is usually safe. Sedation and bradycardia are unrelated effects.
Q236. Answer: B
Explanation: Benzocaine can cause methemoglobinemia in infants if absorbed orally from nipple application. Lidocaine and lanolin are safer for local pain management.
Q237. Answer: B
Explanation: Sulfonamides in TMP-SMX displace bilirubin from albumin, causing kernicterus in neonates. Erythromycin and cephalexin are safe alternatives for lactating mothers.
Q238. Answer: A
Explanation: Sertraline remains the preferred antidepressant due to minimal transfer and low infant plasma levels. Paroxetine and fluoxetine cause more sedation or accumulation.
Q239. Answer: A
Explanation: Dioxins are persistent organic pollutants that concentrate in milk fat, potentially disrupting hormone balance. Nitrates affect oxygenation, not endocrine function. Iron is an essential nutrient.
Q240. Answer: A
Explanation: Drugs with low protein binding, high lipid solubility, and small molecular size cross into milk readily. Molecular weight alone is insufficient; these combined properties determine milk transfer efficiency.
Q241. Answer: C
Explanation: Mastitis requires continued milk removal to prevent abscess formation and appropriate antibiotics targeting S. aureus or MRSA when indicated. Breastfeeding promotes drainage and healing rather than worsening infection.
Q242. Answer: B

Explanation: Plugged ducts typically result from inadequate milk removal, tight clothing, or abrupt feeding schedule changes. Regular, complete breast drainage and avoiding compression help prevent recurrence and mastitis progression.

Q243. Answer: B

Explanation: Breast abscess follows unresolved mastitis with pus collection. Management includes drainage and antibiotics. Milk from the unaffected breast should continue to maintain supply and infant nutrition.

Q244. Answer: A

Explanation: Candidiasis produces deep burning pain during and after feeding, often with shiny nipples and infant oral thrush. Antifungal therapy for both mother and infant is essential to prevent reinfection.

Q245. Answer: B

Explanation: Abscesses require drainage, often by needle aspiration or incision. Continued milk removal promotes healing. Milk from the infected breast may be discarded until antibiotics and drainage control infection.

Q246. Answer: C

Explanation: A milk bleb is a small, blocked nipple pore appearing as a white or yellow blister causing sharp localized pain. Warm compresses and gentle expression resolve blockage.

Q247. Answer: C

Explanation: HIV is a contraindication in high-resource settings with safe formula alternatives. Transmission risk outweighs benefits. In low-resource areas, exclusive breastfeeding may still be recommended per WHO guidance.

Q248. Answer: B

Explanation: Breast milk jaundice appears in healthy infants after the first week, linked to milk factors delaying bilirubin conjugation. It resolves spontaneously with continued breastfeeding.

Q249. Answer: B

Explanation: Poor intake or delayed lactogenesis II leads to increased enterohepatic circulation of bilirubin. Improving feeding frequency and milk transfer corrects the issue without stopping breastfeeding.

Q250. Answer: D

Explanation: Mastitis presents with unilateral erythema, systemic symptoms, and localized tenderness. Prompt antibiotic therapy prevents abscess formation and supports continued breastfeeding.

Q251. Answer: B

Explanation: Benign fibrocystic changes vary with hormonal cycles and cause tenderness premenstrually. They do not contraindicate breastfeeding but require evaluation if masses persist or harden.

Q252. Answer: B

Explanation: Bilious vomiting in newborns is pathologic and may indicate obstruction such as duodenal atresia or malrotation. Immediate evaluation is necessary before oral feeding continues.

Q253. Answer: A

Explanation: Tongue-tie limits tongue extension, impairing latch and effective milk transfer. Frenotomy may improve breastfeeding outcomes when symptoms are significant.

Q254. Answer: A

Explanation: Infants of diabetic mothers often experience hypoglycemia due to high fetal insulin levels. Early, frequent breastfeeding stabilizes glucose levels and reduces supplementation need.

Q255. Answer: A

Explanation: Vasospasm causes ischemic nipple pain triggered by cold exposure or poor latch. Management includes warmth, correcting latch, and sometimes nifedipine in severe cases.

Q256. Answer: B

Explanation: Breast lesions containing active HSV pose transmission risk. Milk expression and feeding from the unaffected breast should continue until lesions heal completely.

Q257. Answer: B
Explanation: Effective feeding is confirmed by audible swallowing, steady stooling, and urination. Frequency alone doesn't ensure milk transfer; assessment of infant output is critical.
Q258. Answer: A
Explanation: A galactocele is a milk retention cyst due to duct obstruction, typically painless and sterile. Aspiration confirms diagnosis; antibiotics are unnecessary unless infected.
Q259. Answer: C
Explanation: Hypothyroidism from Hashimoto disease impairs prolactin responsiveness, reducing milk volume. Proper thyroid hormone replacement restores supply and maternal well-being.
Q260. Answer: A
Explanation: Nipple eczema presents as itchy, crusted lesions; low-potency topical corticosteroids safe for lactation are effective. Avoid strong steroids or unnecessary discontinuation of breastfeeding.
Q261. Answer: A
Explanation: Subclinical mastitis involves inflammatory changes without overt infection. Frequent effective milk removal, warm compresses, and supportive therapy improve ductal drainage and reduce milk sodium levels, preventing progression to acute infection.
Q262. Answer: A
Explanation: Yeast infections transmit easily between mother and infant. Simultaneous antifungal treatment, hygiene reinforcement, and nipple air-drying prevent reinfection. Lactation can safely continue with appropriate management and pain relief.
Q263. Answer: C
Explanation: Mastitis presents with fever, localized pain, erythema, and flu-like symptoms. Blocked ducts typically remain localized without systemic signs. Prompt recognition prevents abscess formation and maintains milk supply.
Q264. Answer: A
Explanation: Advanced mastitis can produce diffuse redness and swelling resembling malignancy. When inflammation fails to resolve with treatment, biopsy and imaging are warranted to rule out inflammatory breast cancer.
Q265. Answer: A
Explanation: Ibuprofen has minimal transfer to milk and offers anti-inflammatory benefits. It reduces pain and swelling without sedation or risk of infant respiratory depression, making it first-line therapy.
Q266. Answer: A
Explanation: Recurrence often stems from milk stasis and nipple trauma. Optimizing latch, breast drainage, and avoiding external pressure support continued lactation while reducing infection risk.
Q267. Answer: C
Explanation: Retained placental tissue sustains progesterone levels, inhibiting milk secretion onset. Medical evaluation and removal restore hormonal balance and milk production.
Q268. Answer: A
Explanation: Green or blue-green milk often results from chlorophyll pigments in diet or vitamin supplements. It is harmless and does not affect milk quality or infant safety.
Q269. Answer: A
Explanation: Codeine metabolizes variably to morphine, and ultra-rapid metabolizers may produce toxic levels in milk. Safer alternatives should be used for pain management during breastfeeding.
Q270. Answer: A
Explanation: Antibiotics such as dicloxacillin or cephalexin are compatible with lactation. The consultant ensures continued milk removal and infant monitoring for mild gut changes.
Q271. Answer: D

Explanation: A galactocele is a benign, non-infectious milk retention cyst often resolving with drainage or gentle aspiration, without the need for antibiotics or surgery.

Q272. Answer: A

Explanation: Low thyroid hormone levels suppress prolactin activity, reducing milk synthesis. Management with appropriate thyroid replacement restores hormonal balance and improves lactation.

Q273. Answer: A

Explanation: Domperidone enhances prolactin release by blocking dopamine receptors. Used under supervision, it aids induced lactation while monitoring for potential cardiac side effects.

Q274. Answer: A

Explanation: Vasospasm causes triphasic color change (white-blue-red) and sharp pain after feeds. Management includes warmth, avoiding cold exposure, and occasionally medication for vascular dilation.

Q275. Answer: D

Explanation: Pseudoephedrine, a decongestant, constricts blood vessels and lowers prolactin levels, decreasing milk production. Lactating mothers should avoid it unless medically necessary.

Q276. Answer: A

Explanation: Fenugreek may enhance supply through mild estrogenic and prolactin-stimulating effects. Clinical results vary, and consultants should discuss safety and potential infant reactions.

Q277. Answer: A

Explanation: Domperidone may prolong QT intervals, posing arrhythmia risk. Cardiac history or interacting medications require caution and medical supervision during galactagogue use.

Q278. Answer: A

Explanation: PCBs, persistent organic pollutants, concentrate in fatty tissues and breast milk. Their presence underscores the importance of environmental regulation and maternal exposure reduction.

Q279. Answer: B

Explanation: Lipid-soluble, low–molecular-weight, weakly basic drugs cross into milk more readily. Protein-bound or ionized compounds remain mostly in maternal plasma, limiting infant exposure.

Q280. Answer: B

Explanation: Ibuprofen has minimal milk transfer and a short half-life, making it preferred for postpartum pain. Codeine and oxycodone may cause infant sedation or respiratory depression.

Q281. Answer: C

Explanation: Amoxicillin has low milk levels and is well tolerated by infants. Tetracycline and chloramphenicol pose risks of bone or marrow toxicity and are avoided during breastfeeding.

Q282. Answer: C

Explanation: Sertraline demonstrates minimal infant serum levels and low adverse effects, making it first-line for lactating mothers with postpartum depression requiring pharmacotherapy.

Q283. Answer: B

Explanation: Estrogen can suppress milk production; progestin-only pills or devices maintain supply and effective contraception. Estrogen-containing methods are delayed until lactation stabilizes.

Q284. Answer: B

Explanation: Agents such as domperidone and metoclopramide enhance prolactin by blocking dopamine receptors. Use requires medical supervision due to potential cardiac or neurologic side effects.

Q285. Answer: A

Explanation: Fenugreek and silymarin (milk thistle) are commonly used natural galactagogues. Evidence for efficacy is limited and quality control varies; safety monitoring is essential.

Q286. Answer: B

Explanation: Pseudoephedrine decreases milk production by vasoconstriction and reduced prolactin response. Decongestants should be avoided in mothers struggling with low supply.

Q287. Answer: B

Explanation: Alcohol peaks in milk within 30–60 minutes and clears with maternal metabolism. Occasional intake is safe once mother feels sober; chronic use impairs letdown and infant development.

Q288. Answer: B

Explanation: Nicotine transfers into milk, causing irritability, tachycardia, and poor sleep in infants. Smoking cessation or nicotine replacement patches away from feeds are preferred.

Q289. Answer: B

Explanation: THC's lipophilicity leads to concentration in milk and prolonged infant exposure. It may impair neurodevelopment; breastfeeding should be discouraged during maternal cannabis use.

Q290. Answer: C

Explanation: Iodine-131 concentrates in milk and infant thyroid; breastfeeding must be stopped permanently for that child. Diagnostic imaging without radioisotopes poses no risk.

Q291. Answer: B

Explanation: Chloramphenicol may cause bone marrow suppression in infants due to immature hepatic metabolism. Safer antibiotic alternatives should be selected for lactating mothers.

Q292. Answer: B

Explanation: Dopamine agonists decrease prolactin secretion, suppressing lactation. They are reserved for medical suppression (e.g., after stillbirth), not routine postpartum management.

Q293. Answer: D

Explanation: Phenobarbital transfers readily into milk and may cause lethargy or feeding difficulties. Monitoring and possible dosage adjustment are required during maternal therapy.

Q294. Answer: B

Explanation: The milk-to-plasma (M/P) ratio quantifies drug concentration in milk relative to maternal plasma. Ratios >1 suggest significant transfer; <1 indicates minimal exposure.

Q295. Answer: A

Explanation: Haloperidol shows low milk transfer compared with atypical agents. Clozapine should be avoided due to agranulocytosis risk. Clinical monitoring remains essential.

Q296. Answer: B

Explanation: References such as LactMed or Breastfeeding and Human Lactation provide current data on drug safety. Many medications are compatible with breastfeeding despite generic warnings.

Q297. Answer: A

Explanation: Sage, parsley, and peppermint in large quantities reduce prolactin and milk volume. Awareness of herbal contraindications is essential for maintaining lactation.

Q298. Answer: B

Explanation: Methyldopa is well-studied and safe for lactation, though fatigue and depression can occur. ACE inhibitors like enalapril are acceptable alternatives, but atenolol may cause infant bradycardia.

Q299. Answer: C

Explanation: Aspirin can cause salicylate toxicity and Reye's syndrome in infants. Acetaminophen and ibuprofen are preferred due to minimal milk transfer and safety profile.

Q300. Answer: C

Explanation: Cytotoxic drugs enter milk and can harm rapidly dividing infant tissues. Breastfeeding must be stopped during chemotherapy and for a safe washout period thereafter.

Questions (301-400)

Q301. Which drug class is most associated with decreased milk production?

A. Beta-blockers
B. Dopamine agonists
C. SSRIs
D. NSAIDs

Q302. Which herbal product may increase bleeding risk in mothers or infants?

A. Fenugreek
B. Ginkgo biloba
C. Milk thistle
D. Goat's rue

Q303. Maternal use of opioids during breastfeeding may result in:

A. Infant lethargy and apnea
B. Improved sleep regulation
C. Increased appetite
D. Decreased bilirubin

Q304. What effect does caffeine have on breastfed infants when consumed in high amounts?

A. Drowsiness
B. Increased irritability and wakefulness
C. Constipation
D. Weight loss inhibition

Q305. Which medication is preferred for treating postpartum depression in lactating mothers?

A. Amitriptyline
B. Sertraline
C. Fluoxetine
D. Bupropion

Q306. What precaution should be taken with maternal metronidazole use?

A. Avoid breastfeeding permanently
B. Interrupt feeding for 12–24 hours after high-dose therapy
C. Continue without adjustment
D. Discard milk for one week

Q307. Herbal tea containing peppermint may:

A. Stimulate letdown reflex
B. Suppress milk supply
C. Prevent mastitis
D. Increase milk fat

Q308. Which medication is safe for treating hypertension postpartum while breastfeeding?

A. Propranolol
B. Atenolol
C. Clonidine
D. Nadolol

Q309. When advising mothers using herbal galactagogues, the consultant should:

A. Encourage unrestricted use
B. Verify purity and evidence for efficacy
C. Dismiss herbal therapies completely
D. Combine multiple herbs for synergy

Q310. Which antibiotic should be avoided due to risk of kernicterus in infants?

A. Amoxicillin
B. Sulfonamides
C. Cephalexin
D. Penicillin
Q311. What principle best minimizes infant drug exposure through milk?
A. Dose immediately before longest infant sleep period
B. Avoid feeding after medication
C. Increase maternal dosage
D. Stop breastfeeding during therapy
Q312. Which medication is preferred for treating postpartum hypertension?
A. Atenolol
B. Nifedipine
C. Propranolol
D. Verapamil
Q313. Which common household chemical is most toxic if ingested by infants through milk?
A. Caffeine
B. Lead
C. Alcohol
D. Fluoride
Q314. What effect can maternal cannabis use have on infants?
A. Enhanced feeding
B. Decreased motor development
C. Improved weight gain
D. Reduced crying
Q315. Which medication is a known galactagogue by dopamine inhibition?
A. Metoclopramide
B. Bromocriptine
C. Lisinopril
D. Atenolol
Q316. Excess iodine exposure in breastfeeding may lead to:
A. Hyperthyroidism in the infant
B. Hypothyroidism in the infant
C. No thyroid effect
D. Dehydration
Q317. Which opioid is contraindicated due to unpredictable metabolism?
A. Morphine
B. Codeine
C. Fentanyl
D. Hydromorphone
Q318. For a mother on anticoagulant therapy, which is safest for breastfeeding?
A. Warfarin
B. Dabigatran
C. Rivaroxaban
D. Heparin
Q319. Chronic alcohol intake during lactation may cause:
A. Hyperactivity
B. Growth retardation and poor motor development
C. Early walking

D. Decreased bilirubin

Q320. A breastfeeding mother taking chemotherapy should:

A. Pump and discard milk
B. Continue feeding with precautions
C. Reduce feeding frequency
D. Alternate breasts

Q321. Which commonly used herb acts as a mild galactagogue?

A. Garlic
B. Echinacea
C. Aloe vera
D. Valerian

Q322. A mother asks about caffeine in chocolate. Consultant advises:

A. Avoid all chocolate
B. Limit to moderate portions
C. Increase intake for energy
D. Substitute with cola

Q323. Which maternal condition may contraindicate use of certain herbal supplements?

A. Asthma
B. Hypertension
C. Hypothyroidism
D. Lactose intolerance

Q324. What is the safest approach for medication counseling in lactation?

A. Evaluate drug class, timing, and infant age
B. Use package inserts only
C. Advise complete cessation
D. Follow online forums

Q325. Which anesthetic is considered compatible with breastfeeding?

A. Halothane
B. Propofol
C. Ether
D. Nitrous oxide

Q326. Which vaccine is contraindicated during lactation?

A. MMR
B. Varicella
C. Smallpox
D. Influenza

Q327. Which drug can cause infant hemolysis in G6PD deficiency?

A. Nitrofurantoin
B. Cephalexin
C. Penicillin
D. Amoxicillin

Q328. The use of diuretics during lactation can:

A. Enhance milk supply
B. Suppress milk production
C. Increase milk fat
D. Improve hydration

Q329. Which thyroid medication is safe during breastfeeding?

A. Methimazole

B. Propylthiouracil
C. Both A and B in low doses
D. Neither A nor B

Q330. What is the mechanism of domperidone as a galactagogue?
A. Inhibits dopamine receptors
B. Stimulates oxytocin release
C. Enhances estrogen receptors
D. Reduces serotonin

Q331. Which antibiotic may stain developing teeth and bones in infants?
A. Tetracycline
B. Amoxicillin
C. Cefalexin
D. Azithromycin

Q332. Which maternal psychiatric drug requires infant monitoring for sedation?
A. Sertraline
B. Diazepam
C. Paroxetine
D. Escitalopram

Q333. Which herbal supplement can cause liver toxicity and should be avoided?
A. Kava
B. Fenugreek
C. Milk thistle
D. Blessed thistle

Q334. Which sedative-hypnotic has minimal milk transfer and can be used short-term?
A. Zolpidem
B. Diazepam
C. Barbiturate
D. Chloral hydrate

Q335. Which maternal supplement may improve infant DHA status?
A. Omega-3 fatty acids
B. Iron
C. Vitamin C
D. Calcium

Q336. Which topical medication is safe for nipple candidiasis treatment?
A. Miconazole cream
B. Hydrocortisone 2%
C. Terbinafine
D. Salicylic acid

Q337. Which nutrient deficiency can mimic low milk supply symptoms?
A. Iron
B. Vitamin D
C. Iodine
D. Zinc

Q338. Maternal use of pseudoephedrine typically causes:
A. Increased milk flow
B. Decreased milk production
C. Enhanced letdown
D. Reduced engorgement only

Q339. What is the most critical safety consideration when prescribing any medication to lactating women?
A. Milk-to-plasma ratio
B. Maternal tolerance
C. Cost of medication
D. Convenience of dosing
Q340. Which factor increases risk of infant sedation from maternal medications?
A. Older infant age
B. Preterm birth and immature metabolism
C. Short maternal dosing interval
D. Use of topical medication
Q341. A lactating mother on long-term antiepileptic therapy should ensure:
A. Routine infant serum level monitoring
B. Discontinuation of breastfeeding
C. Dose reduction below therapeutic level
D. Switching to herbal treatment
Q342. Maternal use of lithium during breastfeeding requires:
A. No monitoring needed
B. Regular infant thyroid and renal function checks
C. Complete weaning
D. Increased maternal dosage
Q343. Which vitamin in excess can cause toxicity in breastfed infants?
A. Vitamin C
B. Vitamin D
C. Vitamin E
D. Vitamin K
Q344. Which factor decreases drug passage into breast milk?
A. High lipid solubility
B. High protein binding
C. Low molecular weight
D. Alkaline pH
Q345. Which antidepressant carries higher infant exposure due to long half-life?
A. Sertraline
B. Venlafaxine
C. Citalopram
D. Fluoxetine
Q346. Maternal use of diuretics postpartum should be:
A. Encouraged for faster recovery
B. Avoided if breastfeeding continuation is desired
C. Increased during engorgement
D. Combined with galactagogues
Q347. Which environmental toxin poses the greatest risk to infant neurodevelopment via breast milk?
A. BPA
B. Lead
C. Ethanol
D. Fluoride
Q348. Which maternal medication class can cause infant hypoglycemia?
A. Beta-blockers

B. ACE inhibitors
C. Calcium channel blockers
D. NSAIDs

Q349. Herbal use of fennel tea for lactation should be approached with:
A. Encouragement and free use
B. Caution due to possible estrogenic effects
C. Avoidance only after 6 months
D. Combination with fenugreek

Q350. Maternal cannabis use can result in:
A. Increased infant appetite
B. Neurobehavioral delays and sedation
C. Faster infant growth
D. Enhanced milk flow

Q351. What is the safest method for managing allergic rhinitis in lactating women?
A. First-generation antihistamines
B. Second-generation antihistamines
C. Nasal decongestants
D. Oral steroids

Q352. Maternal exposure to mercury most commonly occurs through:
A. Inhalation of gasoline fumes
B. Contact with plastics
C. Drinking water
D. Fish consumption

Q353. What should be advised for lactating mothers using nicotine replacement therapy (NRT)?
A. Avoid all NRT
B. Use NRT immediately after nursing
C. Increase patch dose
D. Smoke concurrently

Q354. What is the primary concern with maternal use of opioids like oxycodone?
A. Infant dehydration
B. Infant respiratory depression
C. Maternal engorgement
D. Rapid milk letdown

Q355. Which antidepressant may cause more infant irritability and sleep disturbance?
A. Sertraline
B. Fluoxetine
C. Escitalopram
D. Duloxetine

Q356. Which maternal habit most reduces milk ejection reflex?
A. High fluid intake
B. Cigarette smoking
C. High protein diet
D. Sleep deprivation

Q357. For a mother on necessary radioactive therapy, breastfeeding can resume when:
A. The isotope has decayed to safe levels
B. Infant reaches six months
C. The mother feels well
D. Milk appears clear

Q358. Which commonly used herbal supplement may cause allergic reactions or hypoglycemia in infants?
A. Fenugreek
B. Milk thistle
C. Blessed thistle
D. Alfalfa
Q359. What is the recommended approach for pain control after cesarean in breastfeeding women?
A. Avoid all medications
B. Rely solely on opioids
C. Use multimodal non-opioid analgesia
D. Delay feeding for 24 hours
Q360. A lactation consultant summarizing pharmacologic safety advises:
A. Most medications are compatible with breastfeeding when evaluated correctly
B. Breastfeeding must stop with any medication
C. Only herbal remedies are safe
D. Drug safety is identical for all infants
Q361. A mother expresses guilt about supplementing her baby with formula after a difficult birth. Which initial approach best supports her psychosocial needs?
A. Emphasize exclusive breastfeeding goals
B. Validate her feelings and explore barriers
C. Correct her misconceptions immediately
D. Recommend discontinuing formula use
Q362. Which factor most influences a mother's breastfeeding confidence in collectivist cultures?
A. Hospital policies
B. Peer and family approval
C. Online educational resources
D. Maternal age
Q363. During counseling, a mother reports postpartum sadness and anxiety about milk supply. What is the IBCLC's best role?
A. Prescribe antidepressants
B. Refer to mental health support while addressing lactation
C. Encourage longer feeding sessions
D. Ignore mood until supply stabilizes
Q364. Which approach demonstrates cultural humility during lactation support?
A. Applying uniform feeding recommendations
B. Correcting traditional beliefs directly
C. Avoiding cultural topics to prevent offense
D. Asking open-ended questions about family practices
Q365. A mother's mother-in-law insists on early supplementation. The IBCLC's best strategy is to:
A. Provide private education only to the mother
B. Involve the family in discussing evidence-based feeding
C. Correct the relative publicly
D. Ignore the family dynamic
Q366. What psychosocial factor most predicts early breastfeeding cessation in working mothers?
A. Perceived employer support
B. Number of children
C. Type of infant feeding class attended
D. Maternal BMI

Q367. Which statement best represents the principle of responsive feeding?
A. Feeding by strict schedule regardless of cues
B. Observing infant hunger and satiety signals
C. Limiting duration to control milk intake
D. Prioritizing parental convenience
Q368. A parent expresses discomfort with public breastfeeding due to cultural stigma. Which IBCLC response is most supportive?
A. Discuss legal rights and public norms
B. Suggest formula feeding outdoors
C. Encourage confrontation with critics
D. Avoid discussing public feeding
Q369. When counseling a mother facing intimate partner violence, what should the IBCLC prioritize?
A. Safety assessment and referral to appropriate services
B. Encouraging co-feeding for bonding
C. Ignoring family conflict
D. Discussing advanced pumping techniques
Q370. Which sociocultural barrier most limits exclusive breastfeeding in urbanized settings?
A. Traditional beliefs in herbal supplements
B. Marketing of breastmilk substitutes
C. High parity
D. Limited maternal education
Q371. A teenage mother doubts her capability to breastfeed. The consultant should first:
A. Provide peer role models and supportive education
B. Correct technical errors immediately
C. Delay sessions until maturity improves
D. Focus on dietary counseling only
Q372. Which family structure factor most strengthens breastfeeding continuity?
A. Partner involvement and shared understanding
B. Extended relatives with conflicting advice
C. Absence of family during postpartum period
D. Maternal isolation for rest
Q373. Which statement reflects maternal empowerment in breastfeeding counseling?
A. Encouraging self-directed decision-making
B. Setting rigid feeding goals
C. Minimizing maternal concerns
D. Dictating appropriate techniques
Q374. Which psychological benefit is most consistently linked to exclusive breastfeeding?
A. Faster uterine involution
B. Improved infant speech development
C. Increased maternal bone density
D. Reduced postpartum depression risk
Q375. When a mother declines breastfeeding due to trauma history, what is the IBCLC's first ethical step?
A. Respect decision and offer emotional support
B. Persuade using infant immunity benefits
C. Reframe trauma as minor barrier
D. Challenge avoidance behaviors
Q376. Which community resource best sustains long-term breastfeeding success?

A. Peer support groups
B. Neonatal intensive care units
C. Private medical offices
D. Online retail forums

Q377. What counseling tone most effectively enhances rapport with diverse families?
A. Neutral curiosity and open listening
B. Directive clinical instruction
C. Detached professionalism
D. Overly casual familiarity

Q378. What primary sociological concept underpins breastfeeding as a public health norm?
A. Psychoanalytic motivation
B. Individualistic autonomy
C. Behavioral economics
D. Social learning theory

Q379. Which barrier most affects breastfeeding self-efficacy after cesarean birth?
A. Delayed skin-to-skin contact
B. Surgical scarring appearance
C. Extended hospital stay
D. Visitor restrictions

Q380. What is the most appropriate counseling focus for a mother experiencing breastfeeding-related anxiety?
A. Combine relaxation techniques with feeding guidance
B. Encourage weaning to reduce stress
C. Avoid discussing emotions
D. Focus solely on milk transfer volumes

Q381. When counseling families from collectivist cultures, the consultant should prioritize:
A. Individual independence in feeding choices
B. Family consensus and shared decision-making
C. Rapid correction of misinformation
D. Emphasizing hospital protocols

Q382. Which cultural belief may positively influence breastfeeding initiation?
A. Colostrum as harmful
B. Breastfeeding as divine duty
C. Early herbal supplementation
D. Formula as modern success

Q383. A mother in a multigenerational home experiences pressure to wean early. Effective intervention includes:
A. Providing evidence-based education to all caregivers
B. Limiting information to the mother only
C. Dismissing elder opinions
D. Avoiding household discussion

Q384. Which social factor most influences continued breastfeeding among low-income mothers?
A. Access to peer support and community networks
B. Type of infant formula available
C. Maternal age under 25
D. Hospital birth location

Q385. In multicultural settings, the consultant ensures equity by:
A. Translating materials and confirming comprehension

B. Using complex medical terminology
C. Limiting consultation time
D. Assuming universal literacy

Q386. Which support type best promotes sustained breastfeeding during maternal return to work?
A. Employer-provided pumping space and breaks
B. Partner emotional reassurance only
C. Access to infant formula vouchers
D. Increased postpartum clinic visits

Q387. A mother's anxiety about milk sufficiency is reinforced by social media misinformation. Effective counseling includes:
A. Confronting her online community
B. Advising media avoidance entirely
C. Ignoring misinformation
D. Providing credible lactation resources and reassurance

Q388. The primary determinant of successful peer counselor programs is:
A. Shared experience and cultural similarity
B. Professional certification
C. Hospital affiliation
D. Duration of sessions

Q389. How does partner inclusion during lactation counseling improve outcomes?
A. Reduces perceived maternal isolation and enhances family cooperation
B. Shifts responsibility away from the mother
C. Increases session time inefficiently
D. Minimizes consultant control

Q390. A mother from a culture practicing delayed initiation believes early feeding causes cramps. The best strategy is to:
A. Explore the belief respectfully and provide physiological education
B. Insist on early feeding as hospital policy
C. Ignore her statement
D. Persuade through authority

Q391. Which sociocultural approach most improves breastfeeding exclusivity in refugee populations?
A. Restricting male attendance
B. Standardized Western feeding classes
C. Incentives for formula abstinence
D. Community-led education in native language

Q392. Which policy-level factor most influences national breastfeeding rates?
A. Paid maternity leave duration
B. Hospital parking availability
C. Prenatal vitamin programs
D. Health influencer campaigns

Q393. When a grandmother advises early solid feeding, effective response includes:
A. Respectfully explaining readiness cues and WHO guidelines
B. Discouraging her involvement
C. Agreeing to maintain harmony
D. Providing contradictory instructions

Q394. What communication style most enhances trust with diverse families?
A. Empathetic listening and reflective dialogue
B. Frequent technical corrections

C. Minimal verbal interaction
D. Rapid directive statements

Q395. Which intervention best mitigates social stigma toward breastfeeding in public?
A. Advising cover usage universally
B. Encouraging private feeding only
C. Limiting feeding duration
D. Public health campaigns normalizing lactation

Q396. A mother reports family criticism about frequent nighttime feeding. Supportive guidance includes:
A. Explaining cluster feeding as normal infant behavior
B. Suggesting formula supplementation
C. Recommending longer feeding intervals
D. Avoiding discussion of night care

Q397. Which group intervention most effectively enhances community breastfeeding rates?
A. Peer-led workshops incorporating cultural narratives
B. Exclusive physician lectures
C. Printed leaflets only
D. Anonymous online surveys

Q398. When a client experiences shame after public criticism, the IBCLC should:
A. Reaffirm self-worth and normalize her experience
B. Minimize her feelings to move forward
C. Focus only on technical feeding aspects
D. Advise isolation during feeding

Q399. Which social determinant has the strongest correlation with breastfeeding initiation?
A. Infant gender
B. Parity above three
C. Cesarean delivery rates
D. Maternal education and income level

Q400. In supporting same-sex couples, inclusive care requires:
A. Neutral language and recognition of both parents' roles
B. Assigning a primary mother by default
C. Avoiding discussion of family structure
D. Focusing only on the lactating parent

Answer key and Explanation (301-400)

Q301. Answer: B

Explanation: Dopamine agonists suppress prolactin release, halting lactation. They are used only for suppression when breastfeeding is contraindicated, not for routine postpartum use.

Q302. Answer: B

Explanation: Ginkgo biloba has antiplatelet effects that may cause bleeding complications. Herbal use requires caution and evaluation for interactions with prescribed medications.

Q303. Answer: A

Explanation: Opioids like codeine or oxycodone transfer into milk and can cause sedation or apnea, especially in CYP2D6 ultra-rapid metabolizers. Close monitoring or alternative analgesics are recommended.

Q304. Answer: B

Explanation: Caffeine passes into milk and may cause jitteriness and poor sleep if maternal intake exceeds 300 mg/day. Moderate consumption is considered safe.

Q305. Answer: B

Explanation: Sertraline is preferred for breastfeeding due to low milk levels and minimal infant effects. Fluoxetine has longer half-life and higher infant exposure risk.

Q306. Answer: B

Explanation: Single high doses of metronidazole may necessitate temporary interruption, while standard doses are compatible. Pumping maintains supply during short breaks.

Q307. Answer: B

Explanation: Peppermint oil and teas can decrease milk production when used in large amounts. Herbal remedies should be evaluated for lactation effects before recommendation.

Q308. Answer: A

Explanation: Propranolol has low milk transfer and minimal infant effects. Atenolol and nadolol are excreted in higher amounts and may cause bradycardia or hypotension in infants.

Q309. Answer: B

Explanation: Many herbs lack standardized production or proven benefits. Consultants should guide mothers to use reputable sources and monitor for adverse reactions in both mother and infant.

Q310. Answer: B

Explanation: Sulfonamides displace bilirubin from albumin, risking kernicterus in neonates. Safer alternatives include penicillins and cephalosporins when antibiotics are required.

Q311. Answer: A

Explanation: Timing medication immediately before infant sleep allows partial drug clearance before next feeding, reducing infant exposure while maintaining therapy effectiveness.

Q312. Answer: B

Explanation: Nifedipine is safe, effective, and has low milk transfer. It's commonly used for postpartum blood pressure management without compromising lactation.

Q313. Answer: B

Explanation: Lead exposure from contaminated environments concentrates in breast milk and damages infant neurodevelopment. Environmental assessment and chelation may be necessary for high maternal levels.

Q314. Answer: B

Explanation: THC crosses into milk and accumulates in fat tissues, leading to delayed motor development and potential cognitive effects. Abstinence from cannabis is recommended during breastfeeding.

Q315. Answer: A

Explanation: Metoclopramide enhances prolactin secretion by blocking dopamine receptors. It is used short-term for lactation failure but may cause depression or fatigue.

Q316. Answer: B
Explanation: Excess iodine from maternal supplements or contrast agents suppresses infant thyroid function. Monitoring of maternal intake and infant thyroid status is advised.
Q317. Answer: B
Explanation: Codeine metabolism varies by CYP2D6 genotype, causing toxic morphine levels in infants of ultra-rapid metabolizers. Alternatives like morphine or hydromorphone are safer.
Q318. Answer: D
Explanation: Heparin and low-molecular-weight heparins are large molecules that do not pass into milk. Warfarin is acceptable, but newer agents lack sufficient lactation data.
Q319. Answer: B
Explanation: Chronic alcohol use suppresses oxytocin and prolactin, reducing milk volume and impairing infant growth and motor function. Counseling for alcohol cessation is critical.
Q320. Answer: A
Explanation: Chemotherapy agents are toxic to infants. Milk should be expressed and discarded to maintain supply but never given to the infant until therapy completion and clearance.
Q321. Answer: A
Explanation: Garlic is traditionally believed to enhance milk production and infant feeding interest. Evidence remains limited but suggests safety in dietary amounts.
Q322. Answer: B
Explanation: Chocolate contains caffeine and theobromine. Moderate consumption is safe, but excessive intake can irritate infants, causing restlessness or wakefulness.
Q323. Answer: B
Explanation: Herbs like licorice or ginseng may raise blood pressure. Lactation consultants should screen for maternal conditions before recommending herbal preparations.
Q324. Answer: A
Explanation: Safe pharmacologic practice requires assessing milk transfer, dosing schedule, and infant maturity. Professional resources ensure evidence-based guidance for breastfeeding mothers.
Q325. Answer: B
Explanation: Propofol clears rapidly from plasma and milk, allowing breastfeeding once the mother is fully awake and alert after anesthesia. No interruption is generally necessary.
Q326. Answer: C
Explanation: Smallpox vaccine virus may spread to infants via skin lesions. All other common vaccines are safe and encouraged for lactating mothers.
Q327. Answer: A
Explanation: Nitrofurantoin may trigger hemolytic anemia in infants with G6PD deficiency. Alternative antibiotics should be selected for affected families.
Q328. Answer: B
Explanation: Diuretics reduce plasma volume and prolactin response, suppressing lactation. They should be avoided unless medically necessary and monitored for hydration status.
Q329. Answer: C
Explanation: Both methimazole and PTU are safe in low doses, but methimazole is preferred due to lower hepatotoxicity risk. Monitor infant thyroid function when mothers are on therapy.
Q330. Answer: A
Explanation: Domperidone increases prolactin secretion by dopamine antagonism without crossing the blood-brain barrier extensively, offering fewer neurological side effects than metoclopramide.
Q331. Answer: A
Explanation: Tetracyclines chelate calcium, causing tooth discoloration and bone effects in infants. Their use during lactation is avoided when alternatives exist.

Q332. Answer: B
Explanation: Benzodiazepines like diazepam have long half-lives and may accumulate in infants, leading to sedation. Shorter-acting agents are preferred with close monitoring.
Q333. Answer: A
Explanation: Kava is linked to hepatotoxicity and is not recommended during lactation. Safety and efficacy of herbal products must be confirmed before maternal use.
Q334. Answer: A
Explanation: Zolpidem's short half-life and low milk levels make it acceptable for occasional maternal insomnia. Mothers should avoid bed-sharing after use.
Q335. Answer: A
Explanation: Maternal omega-3 supplementation enhances DHA content in milk, supporting infant neural development. It is recommended for breastfeeding women with low fish intake.
Q336. Answer: A
Explanation: Miconazole effectively treats Candida infections on the nipple and is safe during breastfeeding. It should be wiped off gently before nursing to minimize ingestion.
Q337. Answer: C
Explanation: Iodine deficiency affects thyroid hormone synthesis and lactogenesis, reducing milk production. Adequate iodine intake is essential during lactation.
Q338. Answer: B
Explanation: Pseudoephedrine constricts blood vessels and reduces prolactin, leading to decreased milk volume. Mothers with supply issues should avoid it.
Q339. Answer: A
Explanation: Milk-to-plasma ratio predicts drug transfer to the infant.
Q340. Answer: B
Explanation: Premature infants have immature hepatic and renal systems, leading to slower clearance of drug residues from breast milk. Caution and dosage review are required in these cases.
Q341. Answer: A
Explanation: Monitoring infant serum levels of antiepileptics ensures safety and early detection of sedation or feeding issues while maintaining maternal seizure control and breastfeeding.
Q342. Answer: B
Explanation: Lithium crosses into milk and may cause hypothyroidism or renal effects. If continued, both maternal and infant serum levels and organ functions should be closely monitored.
Q343. Answer: B
Explanation: High maternal vitamin D supplementation leads to hypercalcemia in infants. Safe maternal dosing should not exceed established tolerable limits unless prescribed medically.
Q344. Answer: B
Explanation: Drugs highly bound to plasma proteins remain in maternal circulation, reducing their transfer to milk. This pharmacokinetic property supports safety for lactation use.
Q345. Answer: D
Explanation: Fluoxetine's long half-life and active metabolite norfluoxetine persist in milk, increasing infant serum levels. Sertraline is safer and preferred for breastfeeding mothers.
Q346. Answer: B
Explanation: Diuretics reduce plasma volume and prolactin levels, impairing milk production. They should only be prescribed for clinical indications with lactation monitoring.
Q347. Answer: B
Explanation: Lead accumulates in maternal bone and is mobilized during lactation. Even low levels in milk can harm infant cognition and neurodevelopment, requiring environmental intervention.
Q348. Answer: A

Explanation: Beta-blockers like propranolol or atenolol can lower infant glucose and heart rate. Monitoring is essential, and safer alternatives may be chosen based on risk-benefit analysis.

Q349. Answer: B

Explanation: Fennel contains phytoestrogens that may influence hormone balance and infant intake. Evidence for efficacy is limited, so moderate, short-term use is recommended.

Q350. Answer: B

Explanation: THC's lipophilic nature allows accumulation in infant fat tissues, leading to sedation and developmental delay. Complete abstinence is advised during lactation.

Q351. Answer: B

Explanation: Second-generation antihistamines like loratadine are less sedating and have minimal milk transfer, making them preferable for breastfeeding mothers.

Q352. Answer: D

Explanation: Mercury bioaccumulates in fish; frequent consumption of high-mercury species exposes infants to neurotoxic levels. Advising low-mercury seafood intake supports safe breastfeeding.

Q353. Answer: B

Explanation: NRT is safer than smoking. Timing use after feeding minimizes infant exposure. Gradual dose reduction aids cessation while maintaining breastfeeding safety.

Q354. Answer: B

Explanation: Oxycodone passes readily into milk and can suppress infant respiration and alertness. Safer analgesics should be chosen when possible.

Q355. Answer: B

Explanation: Due to high milk levels and long half-life, fluoxetine increases risk of irritability or colic in infants. Close monitoring is warranted if no alternative is possible.

Q356. Answer: B

Explanation: Nicotine constricts blood vessels and interferes with oxytocin, inhibiting letdown. Smoking cessation enhances milk ejection and infant feeding patterns.

Q357. Answer: A

Explanation: Radioisotopes vary in half-life and milk excretion. Breastfeeding can safely resume once radioactive decay and clearance meet safe exposure thresholds.

Q358. Answer: A

Explanation: Fenugreek may cause maple syrup odor in urine and allergic reactions, especially in families with legume allergies. Monitoring for sensitivity is advised.

Q359. Answer: C

Explanation: Combining NSAIDs and acetaminophen minimizes opioid need while maintaining effective pain relief and supporting early breastfeeding initiation.

Q360. Answer: A

Explanation: Evidence-based pharmacology demonstrates that most maternal medications are compatible with breastfeeding when dosage, timing, and infant maturity are properly considered.

Q361. Answer: B

Explanation: Emotional validation strengthens trust and reduces guilt, creating openness for gradual improvement. Unlike direct correction, this empathetic approach aligns with person-centered lactation care. Options A and D increase stress; C risks defensiveness by disregarding emotional readiness.

Q362. Answer: B

Explanation: Family and community approval directly affect maternal confidence where social norms dominate infant feeding choices. Hospital and media influences are secondary. Age contributes but is less predictive than perceived social acceptance and support.

Q363. Answer: B

Explanation: Lactation consultants must integrate psychosocial screening with referral and ongoing feeding guidance. This dual attention ensures safety and emotional recovery. Ignoring symptoms or changing feeding duration neglects underlying maternal wellbeing.

Q364. Answer: D

Explanation: Open inquiry acknowledges diversity and builds rapport, allowing individualized care. Cultural humility prioritizes learning from the mother's perspective. Avoidance and correction undermine trust, while uniform advice disregards cultural context.

Q365. Answer: B

Explanation: Involving relatives respectfully enhances family buy-in and reduces conflict. Family inclusion acknowledges social influence and builds supportive consensus. Private education or confrontation risks resistance and isolation.

Q366. Answer: A

Explanation: Employer attitudes and workplace accommodations critically determine continuation rates. Supportive environments mitigate stress and maintain milk production. Other factors contribute indirectly but lack consistent predictive power.

Q367. Answer: B

Explanation: Responsive feeding builds trust, self-regulation, and secure attachment by following infant cues. Scheduling disregards physiological needs, and control-based methods disrupt milk regulation and bonding.

Q368. Answer: A

Explanation: Empowering parents with factual, rights-based reassurance fosters confidence and advocacy. Avoidance or confrontation increases distress. Education balances sensitivity with empowerment, reducing shame.

Q369. Answer: A

Explanation: Immediate safety and referral override all other concerns. Lactation guidance follows stabilization. Ignoring danger or focusing on technique violates ethical care and maternal protection standards.

Q370. Answer: B

Explanation: Aggressive formula marketing normalizes bottle-feeding and undermines confidence. Education alone cannot counter pervasive advertising influence. Traditional beliefs have smaller reach in modernized contexts.

Q371. Answer: A

Explanation: Adolescents benefit from relatable support and skill demonstration that build self-efficacy. Technical correction without empathy fails to address insecurity. Delaying or diverting focus impedes confidence growth.

Q372. Answer: A

Explanation: Partner engagement reinforces motivation and reduces perceived burden. Conflicting or absent support undermines sustainability. Emotional availability from partners correlates with longer breastfeeding duration.

Q373. Answer: A

Explanation: Empowerment arises from informed autonomy and shared decision-making. Dictation or rigid standards limit agency, while minimizing concerns diminishes trust. Supportive collaboration builds resilience and adherence.

Q374. Answer: D

Explanation: Exclusive breastfeeding stabilizes oxytocin and prolactin levels, lowering depressive symptoms. Physical benefits exist but are secondary to consistent emotional improvements. Hormonal balance enhances maternal wellbeing.

Q375. Answer: A

Explanation: Respecting autonomy protects psychological safety and dignity. Persuasion or minimizing trauma re-triggers distress. Supportive acceptance fosters healing and possible future reconsideration.

Q376. Answer: A

Explanation: Peer groups offer emotional reinforcement, shared experience, and practical solutions aligned with real-life challenges. Medical offices provide expertise but limited continuity. Online forums lack verified guidance.

Q377. Answer: A

Explanation: Curiosity communicates respect and invites disclosure, key to culturally safe dialogue. Directive or detached tones inhibit openness, while excessive informality risks reduced credibility.

Q378. Answer: D

Explanation: Observational learning drives imitation of modeled behaviors, explaining cultural transmission of breastfeeding. Other frameworks describe individual motivation but lack social propagation emphasis.

Q379. Answer: A

Explanation: Immediate contact promotes hormonal bonding and confidence; delays weaken initiation success. Physical recovery issues are secondary. Early tactile connection restores maternal control and readiness.

Q380. Answer: A

Explanation: Integrating mindfulness with technical instruction addresses physiological and emotional factors concurrently. Avoidance or premature weaning neglects treatable anxiety and disrupts lactation success.

Q381. Answer: B

Explanation: In collectivist contexts, harmony and joint agreement maintain trust and compliance. Promoting shared discussion validates family hierarchy. Insisting on independence or rigid clinical adherence risks cultural alienation and reduced acceptance.

Q382. Answer: B

Explanation: Viewing breastfeeding as sacred reinforces motivation and identity-based adherence. Misbeliefs about colostrum and modern substitutes undermine initiation. Cultural strengths should be leveraged to sustain exclusive feeding.

Q383. Answer: A

Explanation: Family-wide education fosters collective understanding and diminishes generational conflict. Excluding elders or silencing concerns damages relationships and decreases maternal support for continued breastfeeding.

Q384. Answer: A

Explanation: Peer networks compensate for resource gaps, offering emotional and informational reinforcement. Economic or demographic variables alone don't ensure persistence; trusted social systems predict long-term adherence.

Q385. Answer: A

Explanation: Inclusive translation with feedback guarantees informed consent and equitable understanding. Jargon and time limitation create disparities. Literacy assumptions ignore accessibility barriers critical in global lactation care.

Q386. Answer: A

Explanation: Structural supports like designated pumping time and private spaces empower continuation. Emotional or financial factors assist but cannot replace environmental facilitation of milk expression and storage.

Q387. Answer: D

Explanation: Guiding mothers toward verified evidence and reassurance restores confidence without isolation. Blanket avoidance is unrealistic; addressing fears empathetically fosters informed resilience against myths.

Q388. Answer: A

Explanation: Relatability and cultural resonance enhance credibility and participation. Certification and structure help, but emotional identification ensures stronger influence on feeding behaviors and self-efficacy.

Q389. Answer: A

Explanation: Engaging partners validates shared responsibility and fosters supportive home dynamics. It improves adherence through collaborative involvement rather than burden shifting or inefficiency concerns.

Q390. Answer: A

Explanation: Understanding belief origins opens opportunity for education without disrespect. Combining empathy with gentle explanation builds acceptance; strict enforcement fosters opposition and mistrust.

Q391. Answer: D

Explanation: Language and cultural relatability build confidence and accessibility. Western-only or restrictive methods alienate participants. Inclusion transforms community into active partners in infant nutrition goals.

Q392. Answer: A

Explanation: Protected leave enables sustained exclusive feeding and postnatal recovery. Infrastructure and supplementation are secondary. Legislative support correlates directly with duration and initiation success.

Q393. Answer: A

Explanation: Polite education preserves respect and updates generational knowledge. Exclusion or passive agreement maintains misinformation. Balanced dialogue supports maternal authority and continuity of care.

Q394. Answer: A

Explanation: Active empathy and reflection reveal unspoken concerns and foster collaborative partnership. Overcorrection or brevity undermines safety and openness crucial in cross-cultural lactation care.

Q395. Answer: D

Explanation: Broad social normalization shifts community perception, empowering mothers through visibility. Restrictive or concealment-focused advice reinforces stigma and limits breastfeeding freedom.

Q396. Answer: A

Explanation: Clarifying physiological feeding patterns reassures and educates families about newborn needs. Supplementation or scheduling undermines lactation physiology and maternal confidence.

Q397. Answer: A

Explanation: Story-based education resonates culturally and promotes peer modeling. Didactic or impersonal formats lack emotional reinforcement necessary for behavioral change and commitment.

Q398. Answer: A

Explanation: Normalization and reassurance rebuild confidence and resilience. Dismissive or avoidance approaches intensify emotional distress, whereas validation restores agency and coping.

Q399. Answer: D

Explanation: Higher education and socioeconomic stability improve awareness, access, and confidence. Biological or demographic variables have weaker association when social context is controlled.

Q400. Answer: A

Explanation: Affirming diverse roles ensures dignity and equal partnership, essential for trust and shared caregiving. Default assumptions or avoidance marginalize families, reducing engagement and confidence.

Questions (401-500)

Q401. What behavioral factor most predicts breastfeeding duration among first-time mothers?

A. Self-efficacy and confidence level
B. Hospital birth type
C. Infant gender
D. Length of maternity leave

Q402. Which societal pressure most discourages breastfeeding in high-income countries?

A. Return-to-work expectations
B. Family proximity
C. Access to breast pumps
D. Rooming-in hospital policies

Q403. What public health measure best combats misinformation about lactation online?

A. Verified government or NGO digital campaigns
B. Anonymous chat forums
C. Personal testimonials only
D. Banning all lactation discussions

Q404. A mother returning to work reports decreased pumping output. Which primary psychosocial factor may explain this change?

A. Office temperature
B. Pump brand variation
C. Infant weaning interest
D. Stress and reduced relaxation during pumping

Q405. Which behavioral model explains the impact of social influence on lactation behavior?

A. Theory of Planned Behavior
B. Classical Conditioning
C. Maslow's Hierarchy
D. Piaget's Developmental Theory

Q406. Which intervention most effectively reduces disparities in breastfeeding initiation rates?

A. Culturally adapted prenatal education
B. Increasing hospital discharge speed
C. Expanding formula sample distribution
D. Standardizing postpartum visits

Q407. A mother's partner discourages nighttime feeding due to sleep disruption. What is the IBCLC's best course?

A. Educate on normal infant sleep and feeding patterns
B. Advise ignoring partner concerns
C. Recommend bottle substitution
D. Defer discussion until next visit

Q408. Which public campaign message best supports breastfeeding normalization?

A. "Feeding anytime, anywhere is healthy and normal."
B. "Breastfeeding is only for stay-at-home mothers."
C. "Cover yourself for modesty."
D. "Formula is equally ideal."

Q409. A client from a rural area believes breastmilk loses value after six months. Best consultant response is:

A. Ignore the belief

B. Correct her sharply
C. Recommend immediate weaning
D. Share WHO evidence showing continued nutritional benefits

Q410. How does maternal depression influence infant feeding behaviors?
A. Reduces responsiveness to infant cues and feeding consistency
B. Increases milk production
C. Enhances bonding
D. Improves infant appetite

Q411. What community-level factor most predicts sustained breastfeeding?
A. Accessibility of postnatal home visits
B. Urban housing density
C. Regional climate
D. Proximity to retail stores

Q412. When addressing workplace lactation barriers, IBCLCs advocate primarily for:
A. Legally protected break time and private spaces
B. Free infant formula
C. Company-sponsored parenting classes
D. Limiting pumping to lunch breaks

Q413. What belief contributes most to perceived milk insufficiency?
A. Infant gender bias
B. Lack of breast fullness
C. Small maternal breast size
D. Misinterpretation of infant behavior as hunger

Q414. Which behavioral technique supports anxious mothers during feeding sessions?
A. Guided relaxation and deep breathing
B. Timed feeding limitation
C. Avoiding infant eye contact
D. Counting suck frequency

Q415. Which public facility adaptation most encourages breastfeeding inclusivity?
A. Designated comfortable, hygienic feeding areas
B. Restriction to restrooms
C. Mandatory covering policies
D. Paid feeding permits

Q416. A mother from a patriarchal culture defers all feeding decisions to her spouse. IBCLC action should be:
A. Encourage shared but autonomous maternal input
B. Respect silence without comment
C. Engage spouse exclusively
D. Recommend separate sessions

Q417. What messaging best supports inclusive breastfeeding promotion for fathers and partners?
A. Centering only on maternal nutrition
B. Minimizing their involvement
C. Highlighting their vital role in support and care
D. Using gendered stereotypes

Q418. Which intervention addresses both nutrition and emotional bonding effectively?
A. Promoting skin-to-skin contact immediately post-birth
B. Scheduling feeds every three hours
C. Avoiding physical contact after feeding

D. Introducing bottles early
Q419. How can healthcare systems promote societal breastfeeding normalization?
A. Integrating breastfeeding imagery in routine health communication
B. Limiting visual representation to clinical manuals
C. Avoiding mention in mass media
D. Regulating privacy mandates
Q420. What parental factor most enhances success in combination feeding plans?
A. Clear communication and realistic shared expectations
B. Frequent switching between feeding methods
C. Maintaining secrecy about formula use
D. Avoiding professional input
Q421. Which positioning principle ensures optimal milk transfer during breastfeeding?
A. Baby's chin away from the breast
B. Infant's nose level with the nipple
C. Mother leaning backward completely
D. Infant's ear, shoulder, and hip misaligned
Q422. What first-hour action most enhances long-term breastfeeding success?
A. Immediate skin-to-skin and self-attachment
B. Early pacifier introduction
C. Delayed contact until maternal rest
D. Routine swaddling and nursery separation
Q423. A mother experiences nipple pain during feeds. The first step is to:
A. Assess positioning and latch technique
B. Recommend nipple shields immediately
C. Shorten feeding duration
D. Apply lanolin without assessment
Q424. Which feeding cue indicates readiness to latch?
A. Rooting and mouth opening
B. Crying loudly
C. Turning head away
D. Hand fisting with tension
Q425. The most effective intervention for poor weight gain despite frequent feeds is:
A. Increase burping intervals
B. Offer water between feeds
C. Introduce formula immediately
D. Evaluate and improve latch depth
Q426. Which mother–infant position best supports feeding with large breasts?
A. Football (clutch) hold
B. Cradle hold
C. Side-lying with infant below nipple
D. Upright straddle hold
Q427. For infants with weak suck, the IBCLC should recommend:
A. Breast compression to assist flow
B. Decreasing feeding frequency
C. Limiting time at breast
D. Immediate bottle substitution
Q428. What sign confirms effective milk transfer during feeding?
A. Audible swallowing and rhythmic sucking

B. Constant shallow nibbling
C. Cheeks dimpling inward
D. Absence of movement

Q429. What is the primary benefit of biological nurturing positions?
A. Promotes early pacifier use
B. Enforces rigid posture for control
C. Minimizes maternal movement
D. Utilizes gravity for self-attachment and comfort

Q430. A preterm infant tires quickly at the breast. The consultant should:
A. Use paced, partial feeds with expressed milk supplementation
B. Recommend formula exclusively
C. Delay all oral feeds until term
D. Extend sessions indefinitely

Q431. When assisting latch for flat nipples, the best strategy is:
A. Hand-express to evert nipple before latch
B. Apply firm pressure with pump
C. Delay feeds until nipple shape changes
D. Use ice packs pre-feed

Q432. What tool ensures proper latch evaluation objectively?
A. Direct observation of suck–swallow rhythm
B. Maternal nipple color post-feed
C. Weight chart comparison only
D. Duration of feeding

Q433. How can the IBCLC support mothers with back pain during feeding?
A. Avoid addressing comfort issues
B. Shorten feed times drastically
C. Recommend standing while nursing
D. Suggest ergonomic positioning and supportive cushions

Q434. What is the advantage of the side-lying breastfeeding position?
A. Promotes rest for mother and infant while maintaining closeness
B. Reduces bonding cues
C. Restricts milk drainage
D. Encourages shallow latch

Q435. What indicates need for repositioning during breastfeeding?
A. Nipple pain, clicking sounds, or infant frustration
B. Occasional burping
C. Maternal sweating
D. Infant eye contact

Q436. How can an IBCLC optimize milk flow during sleepy infant feeds?
A. Breast compression and tactile stimulation
B. Shortening feeding time
C. Offering pacifier first
D. Cooling the room

Q437. Which position minimizes reflux symptoms in infants?
A. Side-lying flat on back
B. Fully supine feeding
C. Overhead cradle
D. Upright or semi-reclined feeding posture

Q438. A mother reports rapid milk ejection overwhelming her newborn. The IBCLC should recommend:
A. Leaning back or reclined feeding position
B. Increasing compression
C. Switching breasts rapidly
D. Avoiding nursing temporarily
Q439. Which assessment best determines adequate milk transfer in early weeks?
A. Infant weight gain and diaper output trends
B. Maternal breast fullness only
C. Feeding frequency alone
D. Infant crying volume
Q440. What is the key IBCLC intervention for infants refusing the breast?
A. Promote skin-to-skin contact and calm reintroduction
B. Forcing latch repeatedly
C. Prolonged withholding of feeds
D. Offering pacifier substitution
Q441. What guideline ensures hygienic expression and storage of human milk?
A. Mix old and fresh milk freely
B. Boil milk before storage
C. Wash hands, use clean containers, and refrigerate within four hours
D. Use any plastic container available
Q442. Which pumping strategy best maintains milk production for working mothers?
A. Pump every 3–4 hours for 15–20 minutes
B. Pump once daily at night
C. Skip sessions on busy days
D. Alternate breasts weekly
Q443. For mothers with limited refrigeration, safe milk storage involves:
A. Using insulated cooler with ice packs for up to 24 hours
B. Storing milk at room temperature for two days
C. Keeping milk in open containers
D. Freezing immediately after each pump
Q444. When should hand expression be prioritized over mechanical pumping?
A. Early postpartum or when breasts are engorged
B. When returning to full-time work
C. For exclusive long-term use
D. To reduce stimulation
Q445. What indicator shows effective pumping technique?
A. Collapsed tubing during suction
B. Painful pulling and nipple blanching
C. No milk after several sessions
D. Multiple milk sprays followed by steady flow
Q446. When assisting mothers of multiples, the consultant should recommend:
A. Simultaneous double pumping to save time
B. Alternating infants daily
C. Feeding only one infant directly
D. Restricting feeds to daytime
Q447. What intervention minimizes nipple trauma during pumping?
A. Correct flange size and moderate suction setting
B. High vacuum pressure for faster output

C. Pumping dry breasts
D. Extending sessions indefinitely

Q448. When supplementing with expressed milk, the preferred method is:
A. Cup or spoon feeding
B. Fast-flow bottle nipples
C. Syringe directly to mouth
D. Nipple shield without supervision

Q449. Which pumping practice optimizes oxytocin response?
A. Pumping in noisy environments
B. Rapid suction cycles from the start
C. Viewing baby photos or gentle breast massage before expression
D. Using cold compresses pre-session

Q450. What method supports milk supply during temporary maternal illness?
A. Continue pumping/feeding frequently with hygiene measures
B. Suspend all feeding until full recovery
C. Discard all expressed milk
D. Substitute with cow's milk

Q451. Which storage guideline ensures nutrient preservation after thawing frozen milk?
A. Use within 24 hours and avoid refreezing
B. Reheat repeatedly
C. Keep at room temperature all day
D. Refreeze leftovers

Q452. What is the best intervention for slow milk expression?
A. Gentle breast massage and warm compress pre-session
B. Increasing suction beyond comfort
C. Decreasing pumping frequency
D. Cooling the breast tissue

Q453. How should expressed milk from multiple sessions be combined safely?
A. Combine old and new milk after 24 hours
B. Mix immediately regardless of temperature
C. Add warm milk to cold directly
D. Cool fresh milk first before mixing with refrigerated milk

Q454. A mother uses a hand pump causing nipple blanching. Appropriate adjustment is:
A. Reduce vacuum pressure and ensure proper alignment
B. Increase frequency with same pressure
C. Extend duration to compensate
D. Apply lotion to nipple after each session

Q455. Which practice prevents oversupply when pumping for donation?
A. Gradually taper expression frequency
B. Maintain maximum pumping output
C. Sudden cessation of all pumping
D. Limit hydration

Q456. What supplementation tool minimizes interference with breastfeeding?
A. Supplemental nursing system (SNS) at the breast
B. Wide-neck fast-flow bottle
C. Pacifier pre-feed
D. Spoon-feeding exclusively

Q457. To prevent bacterial contamination of expressed milk, the IBCLC advises:

A. Air-drying inside sealed containers
B. Rinsing with cold water only
C. Cleaning once daily
D. Washing pump parts with hot, soapy water after each use

Q458. A mother returning to shift work struggles with nocturnal expression. Recommended strategy is:
A. Align pumping schedule to infant feeding pattern
B. Skip nighttime pumping entirely
C. Double pumping before sleep only
D. Replace sessions with hydration alone

Q459. Which expression pattern suits mothers with oversupply and leaking?
A. Block pumping, alternating sides every 3–4 hours
B. Pump continuously every hour
C. Express minimally once daily
D. Stop pumping entirely

Q460. What best supports emotional adjustment during long-term milk expression?
A. Encouraging rest, self-care, and realistic expectations
B. Ignoring fatigue and focusing on volume
C. Comparing yields with others
D. Pumping despite exhaustion

Q461. A mother with postpartum depression reports difficulty bonding during feeds. The IBCLC's best action is to:
A. Ignore emotional state
B. Focus on pumping output alone
C. Delay feeding until mood improves
D. Encourage skin-to-skin contact and refer for psychological support

Q462. A father expresses concern about his partner's fatigue from frequent nighttime feeds. The consultant should:
A. Suggest shared caregiving and night assistance with expressed milk
B. Recommend formula to let her sleep
C. Advise separation for rest
D. Ignore paternal involvement

Q463. An anxious mother reports pain despite adequate latch. What should the IBCLC assess first?
A. Maternal muscle tension and anxiety during feeds
B. Pump calibration
C. Infant reflux
D. Feeding duration

Q464. A client relactating after adoption experiences discouragement. Which support method is optimal?
A. Celebrate incremental progress and encourage realistic milestones
B. Compare to biological mothers
C. Demand exclusive feeding immediately
D. Limit expression sessions

Q465. An infant with reflux struggles during rapid let-down. Which position is most suitable?
A. Cradle with downward tilt
B. Flat supine feeding
C. Upright or laid-back breastfeeding position
D. Football hold with infant facing upward

Q466. A mother expresses embarrassment breastfeeding at family gatherings. Effective IBCLC intervention is to:
A. Normalize breastfeeding and discuss discretion techniques if desired
B. Advise formula use publicly
C. Suggest isolation during visits
D. Encourage ignoring feelings
Q467. After returning to work, a mother reports declining output and emotional exhaustion. Optimal approach:
A. Adjust pumping schedule, assess workplace stress, and offer self-care support
B. Prescribe herbal galactagogues immediately
C. Recommend reducing hydration
D. Ignore emotional factors
Q468. When a mother with past trauma resists physical touch during feeds, the IBCLC should:
A. Prioritize consent, create safe environment, and adapt techniques
B. Proceed with physical correction
C. Assume she will adjust over time
D. Insist on skin-to-skin
Q469. A mother of twins feels unequal feeding success. The consultant's first step:
A. Focus on output comparison
B. Recommend weaning one infant
C. Encourage bottle preference
D. Evaluate positioning and emotional balance during tandem sessions
Q470. A grandmother questions colostrum feeding. IBCLC response:
A. Educate gently on colostrum's immune benefits
B. Ignore her involvement
C. Dismiss belief harshly
D. Provide written policy only
Q471. During pumping consult, a mother breaks down about body image changes. IBCLC should:
A. Offer empathetic listening and reinforce body's functionality
B. Divert focus solely to technique
C. Advise cosmetic correction
D. Ignore emotional distress
Q472. A newborn refuses breast after NICU stay. The best reintroduction method is:
A. Skin-to-skin sessions and non-stressful exposure
B. Prolonged forced attempts
C. Continuous bottle-only feeds
D. Ignoring feeding cues
Q473. An overanxious parent records every feed obsessively. The IBCLC's supportive strategy:
A. Remove feeding records entirely
B. Encourage constant data entry
C. Simplify tracking and focus on bonding
D. Ignore anxiety
Q474. In cross-cultural sessions, which behavior demonstrates respect and professionalism?
A. Asking permission before touching mother or infant
B. Assuming consent to adjust latch physically
C. Avoiding communication through interpreter
D. Correcting beliefs immediately
Q475. Which practice best integrates emotional reassurance during technique correction?

A. Praise efforts, then guide improvement constructively
B. Focus solely on technical error
C. Replace hands-on support with lecture
D. Correct abruptly without feedback

Q476. A mother expresses guilt over partial formula use. The IBCLC's best response:
A. Affirm continued breastfeeding benefits and support dual feeding
B. Urge exclusive breastfeeding immediately
C. Warn about harm
D. Avoid the topic

Q477. What interdisciplinary collaboration benefits mothers with postpartum anxiety?
A. Social media peer reliance
B. Exclusive lactation follow-up only
C. Delegation to family
D. Partnership with mental health professionals

Q478. A partner expresses frustration about feeding frequency. Effective IBCLC approach:
A. Educate on infant developmental feeding patterns
B. Suggest bottle supplementation immediately
C. Ignore partner questions
D. Encourage shorter feeds

Q479. Which method combines technique improvement and maternal confidence enhancement?
A. Hands-on guidance with verbal encouragement
B. Silent demonstration without feedback
C. Written handouts only
D. Correction via third party

Q480. A mother coping with grief struggles to maintain supply. The IBCLC's primary goal:
A. Provide emotional support and maintain gentle expression schedule
B. Enforce strict feeding targets
C. Ignore emotional context
D. Suspend lactation care

Q481. A lactation consultant observes a mother with nipple pain during feeding. The infant's chin is not touching the breast and there are audible clicking sounds. What is the most likely issue?
A. Rapid letdown
B. Poor latch and positioning
C. Flat nipples
D. Oversupply

Q482. A new mother reports her baby feeds for long periods but seems unsatisfied. Assessment reveals shallow latch and low milk transfer. Which initial intervention is most appropriate?
A. Increase feeding intervals
B. Recommend nipple shield
C. Reposition for deeper latch
D. Supplement with formula

Q483. A consultant evaluates milk transfer using pre- and post-feeding weights. What best describes this method?
A. Clinical observation technique
B. Indirect measure of intake
C. Direct measure of intake
D. Lactogenesis II assessment

Q484. When teaching hand expression to a postpartum mother, what principle should be emphasized?

A. Firm, quick squeezing motions
B. Gentle rhythmic compression behind are休息ola
C. Pulling nipple forward repeatedly
D. Rotating pressure around nipple tip

Q485. During an inpatient consult, a mother recovering from cesarean birth struggles to position her infant comfortably. What is the best recommendation?
A. Side-lying or football hold
B. Upright cradle hold
C. Prone tummy position
D. Standing assisted latch

Q486. A consultant assists a mother expressing milk for a NICU infant. She asks about ideal storage temperature for 24-hour use. What is correct?
A. 4°C (39°F)
B. 15°C (59°F)
C. 25°C (77°F)
D. 0°C (32°F)

Q487. A mother uses an electric breast pump but experiences nipple soreness and swelling post-session. What adjustment should the consultant recommend first?
A. Decrease suction level
B. Pump longer sessions
C. Apply warm compress afterward
D. Use smaller flange

Q488. Which finding best indicates adequate infant milk transfer during breastfeeding?
A. Mother feels fullness post-feed
B. Infant remains drowsy post-feed
C. Audible swallowing and relaxed tone
D. Breast appears engorged afterward

Q489. A consultant observes excessive maternal nipple blanching post-feed. What is the most probable cause?
A. Vasospasm due to shallow latch
B. Rapid letdown reflex
C. Blocked ducts
D. Infection

Q490. While coaching a family on tandem nursing, which core principle should guide lactation advice?
A. Always nurse older child first
B. Alternate breasts between children daily
C. Prioritize newborn feeding needs
D. Limit nursing sessions per child

Q491. A consultant observes a sleepy infant who often falls asleep at the breast after only a few minutes. What should be assessed first?
A. Maternal diet
B. Infant feeding cues and positioning
C. Maternal nipple shape
D. Infant age only

Q492. A postpartum client reports burning nipple pain during feeding that persists afterward. What is the most likely cause?
A. Candidal infection
B. Vasospasm

C. Trauma from pump flange
D. Blocked duct

Q493. A mother is instructed to use breast compressions during feeding. What is the goal of this technique?

A. Reduce engorgement
B. Enhance milk flow and transfer
C. Prevent leaking
D. Stimulate nipple sensitivity

Q494. During follow-up, a consultant notes maternal breasts remain firm after feeding. What is the likely problem?

A. Ineffective milk removal
B. Overproduction
C. Plugged duct
D. Hormonal suppression

Q495. A baby exhibits gagging and choking shortly after letdown. What is the most suitable intervention?

A. Reclined feeding position
B. Pump to empty both breasts before feeding
C. Restrict feeding duration
D. Use nipple shield immediately

Q496. What feature distinguishes nutritive from non-nutritive sucking?

A. Rhythmic swallowing during nutritive phase
B. Constant jaw movement with no pause
C. Brief bursts followed by silence
D. No swallowing sounds at any time

Q497. A consultant notes an infant repeatedly unlatching. Which adjustment should be tried first?

A. Reposition mother and infant for chin contact
B. Introduce bottle supplementation
C. Use pacifier between feeds
D. Apply nipple ointment

Q498. During expression teaching, which advice supports oxytocin release?

A. Express on rigid schedule only
B. Apply high pump suction
C. Avoid skin contact
D. Relax, massage, and visualize baby before expressing

Q499. A consultant observes the baby has a recessed chin. What modification can assist feeding?

A. Slight breast shaping and asymmetrical latch
B. Nipple shield immediate use
C. Upright sitting only
D. Extended feeding intervals

Q500. Which action best supports continuity of care when transferring clients to another IBCLC?

A. Provide complete documentation and care summary
B. Send verbal message only
C. Retain notes privately
D. Allow client to explain history

Answer key and Explanation (401-500)

Q401. Answer: A

Explanation: Maternal confidence directly influences perseverance and perceived control during early challenges. Birth setting and infant variables have secondary influence. Empowering self-efficacy through education and validation enhances duration and satisfaction.

Q402. Answer: A

Explanation: Workplace reintegration pressure shortens exclusive feeding periods by limiting flexibility. Family support and hospital practices mitigate barriers but cannot offset cultural prioritization of productivity over caregiving.

Q403. Answer: A

Explanation: Evidence-based digital outreach ensures consistency and credibility, counteracting myths effectively. Unregulated peer content perpetuates confusion. Prohibition reduces accessibility to reliable education and damages awareness.

Q404. Answer: D

Explanation: Psychological stress suppresses oxytocin release, limiting let-down reflex and output. Equipment differences or environmental factors exert minimal influence compared to emotional state and privacy level.

Q405. Answer: A

Explanation: The Theory of Planned Behavior emphasizes social norms and perceived control in health-related decisions. Other models explore learning or development but don't directly predict maternal feeding behavior changes.

Q406. Answer: A

Explanation: Tailored prenatal instruction builds cultural trust and addresses unique community beliefs. Generic programs overlook barriers. Formula marketing or premature discharge reduces preparation and support continuity.

Q407. Answer: A

Explanation: Teaching family about physiology normalizes expectations and prevents conflict. Dismissal or delay fosters resentment and misinformation. Shared understanding enhances family cooperation and sustainability.

Q408. Answer: A

Explanation: Normalization messages dismantle stigma by affirming inclusivity and health benefits. Restrictive or comparative phrasing creates division or shame, weakening public acceptance and policy advocacy.

Q409. Answer: D

Explanation: Respectful explanation supported by global evidence reassures while honoring cultural learning. Confrontation discourages dialogue. WHO standards affirm breastfeeding through two years and beyond for optimal outcomes.

Q410. Answer: A

Explanation: Depression impairs sensitivity and timing, disrupting feeding rhythm and attachment. Physiological or appetite changes are secondary consequences. Addressing mood stabilizes dyadic interactions and feeding success.

Q411. Answer: A

Explanation: Ongoing community follow-up provides reassurance and early intervention. Structural or environmental factors matter less than continued personal connection and accessible support networks.

Q412. Answer: A

Explanation: Legal protection ensures equitable opportunity and sustained milk supply. Supplementary measures offer partial aid but without mandated accommodation, mothers face persistent workplace discrimination and decline.

Q413. Answer: D

Explanation: Misreading normal infant cluster feeding as starvation fuels insecurity. Physical appearance or size doesn't correlate with production. Clarifying developmental feeding cycles restores confidence and continuation.

Q414. Answer: A

Explanation: Relaxation mitigates stress-induced letdown inhibition, stabilizing flow and mood. Mechanical monitoring or avoidance heightens tension and undermines positive bonding during feeding.

Q415. Answer: A

Explanation: Clean, accessible spaces validate mothers' rights and comfort without imposing isolation. Restrictive or fee-based systems stigmatize and discourage public feeding, reducing visibility and equality.

Q416. Answer: A

Explanation: Empowering maternal voice while maintaining family harmony promotes equality and informed decision-making. Ignoring imbalance sustains disempowerment; exclusive spousal focus reinforces hierarchy.

Q417. Answer: C

Explanation: Recognizing shared caregiving strengthens emotional bonds and family stability. Marginalization or gender bias alienates partners and limits advocacy potential within family systems.

Q418. Answer: A

Explanation: Skin-to-skin synchronizes physiological regulation and attachment, enhancing milk ejection and parental attunement. Structured scheduling and early bottles interrupt natural rhythms critical for bonding.

Q419. Answer: A

Explanation: Visibility in media reframes breastfeeding as standard, encouraging acceptance. Restrictive or clinical-only portrayals maintain stigma and fail to normalize daily public feeding behavior.

Q420. Answer: A

Explanation: Transparency and planning prevent guilt and inconsistency, sustaining infant nutrition and bonding. Concealment or erratic changes create confusion and stress, undermining both techniques and confidence.

Q421. Answer: B

Explanation: Aligning the infant's nose with the nipple promotes effective latch depth and airway protection. Chin contact and body alignment support suction mechanics. Poor alignment or extreme reclining reduces milk transfer efficiency.

Q422. Answer: A

Explanation: Early skin contact activates feeding reflexes and hormonal priming, ensuring effective early latch and maternal bonding. Delays or artificial soothing interrupt natural feeding initiation and hormonal cascade.

Q423. Answer: A

Explanation: Observing positioning identifies root causes such as shallow latch or misalignment. Symptomatic treatments alone neglect underlying mechanical issues, prolonging discomfort and risking nipple trauma.

Q424. Answer: A

Explanation: Rooting and open-mouth behavior precede distress and signal early hunger. Late cues like crying or tensing indicate missed opportunity. Recognizing early cues maintains calm, effective feeding sessions.

Q425. Answer: D

Explanation: Ineffective latch impedes milk transfer even with frequent attempts. Hydration and formula aren't first-line unless supply proven low. Proper latch restores intake and growth naturally.

Q426. Answer: A

Explanation: The football hold offers visibility and control, reducing pressure on the breast and airway. Other positions may obscure latch quality or hinder alignment for mothers with fuller anatomy.

Q427. Answer: A

Explanation: Gentle compression increases flow and encourages active sucking, strengthening feeding ability. Limiting sessions or substituting early prevents skill development and reduces supply stimulus.

Q428. Answer: A

Explanation: Audible swallows show coordinated suck–swallow–breathe pattern and flow. Shallow or dimpled motion suggests poor seal and inadequate transfer. Stillness signals fatigue or weak suck reflex.

Q429. Answer: D

Explanation: Reclined positions enable infant-led rooting via innate reflexes. Relaxed posture enhances oxytocin release and reduces strain. Rigid control methods impede natural behavioral synchronization.

Q430. Answer: A

Explanation: Combining direct feeding with expressed supplementation maintains nutrition and skill practice. Full delay or overexertion risks fatigue and aspiration. Tailored pacing supports maturation and success.

Q431. Answer: A

Explanation: Gentle expression promotes protrusion and stimulates flow, facilitating latch. Pump pressure or delay hinders progress and frustrates infant readiness. Cold constricts tissue, worsening inversion.

Q432. Answer: A

Explanation: Observing coordinated rhythm and audible swallowing provides real-time functional assessment. Weight and color are secondary indicators; timing alone cannot determine adequacy or transfer efficiency.

Q433. Answer: D

Explanation: Physical comfort ensures relaxation and oxytocin release, improving let-down. Ignoring ergonomics perpetuates pain and early weaning. Position aids sustain endurance and posture health.

Q434. Answer: A

Explanation: Side-lying supports recovery, relaxation, and sustained contact without strain. Proper alignment prevents shallow latch. Misuse or fear of sleep association should be addressed through safe co-positioning.

Q435. Answer: A

Explanation: Audible clicking and discomfort reveal air leakage and shallow latch requiring correction. Burping and contact are normal. Persistent misalignment diminishes transfer and nipple integrity.

Q436. Answer: A

Explanation: Compression maintains flow and alertness, enhancing intake without overexertion. Pacifiers or shortened sessions decrease stimulation. Cold environments lower arousal and oxytocin response.

Q437. Answer: D

Explanation: Upright positioning uses gravity to prevent regurgitation and discomfort. Flat feeding increases reflux and aspiration risk. Proper angling promotes digestion and comfort post-feed.

Q438. Answer: A

Explanation: Reclined positioning slows gravity flow and gives infant better control. Compression or avoidance worsen symptoms or reduce supply. Adjusting posture balances let-down intensity safely.

Q439. Answer: A

Explanation: Weight and output provide measurable indicators of intake effectiveness. Isolated cues like crying or fullness are unreliable. Consistent monitoring ensures accurate progress evaluation.

Q440. Answer: A

Explanation: Rebuilding positive association through calm skin contact resets reflexive comfort and trust. Forcing or withholding creates aversion. Gradual re-exposure fosters renewed acceptance and success.

Q441. Answer: C

Explanation: Hand hygiene and timely refrigeration prevent bacterial growth and nutrient degradation. Boiling destroys immunologic factors; random mixing and non-sterile storage risk contamination and loss of quality.

Q442. Answer: A

Explanation: Regular expression mimics feeding frequency, sustaining prolactin response and supply stability. Skipping or infrequent sessions suppresses output, while uneven alternation causes engorgement and discomfort.

Q443. Answer: A

Explanation: Portable cooling preserves freshness during transport and aligns with WHO safety guidelines. Room temperature and open storage increase bacterial risk, while constant freezing complicates rotation and thawing.

Q444. Answer: A

Explanation: Hand expression aids early milk removal and relieves engorgement gently. It supports oxytocin reflex naturally. Exclusive mechanical use suits established supply; manual method ensures comfort and responsiveness.

Q445. Answer: D

Explanation: Rhythmic sprays signify proper stimulation and compression sequence. Pain and blanching reflect excessive vacuum. Absence of flow or tubing collapse indicates mechanical malfunction or misfit.

Q446. Answer: A

Explanation: Double pumping increases oxytocin peaks, efficiency, and milk volume while reducing maternal fatigue. Alternation or restriction impairs supply and bonding balance between infants.

Q447. Answer: A

Explanation: Proper flange fit prevents friction, and moderate suction preserves comfort and tissue integrity. Excessive vacuum or dry pumping damages epithelium and discourages continuation.

Q448. Answer: A

Explanation: Alternative methods reduce nipple confusion and preserve breastfeeding coordination. Fast-flow bottles interfere with suck rhythm. Unmonitored shields or syringes risk aspiration or ineffective feeding.

Q449. Answer: C

Explanation: Emotional connection and tactile stimulation trigger oxytocin, facilitating let-down. Stressful or cold conditions suppress hormonal reflexes, reducing yield and comfort.

Q450. Answer: A

Explanation: Frequent removal maintains supply while proper hygiene prevents pathogen transfer. Temporary cessation reduces prolactin stimulus and increases engorgement risk. Safe continuation sustains flow and immunity.

Q451. Answer: A

Explanation: Thawed milk retains antibodies only if used promptly under refrigeration. Reheating or refreezing degrades components and raises contamination risk. Controlled temperature management is essential.

Q452. Answer: A

Explanation: Warmth and massage stimulate let-down reflex by enhancing circulation. Excess suction or reduced frequency worsens flow issues. Cooling constricts ducts and reduces hormonal response.

Q453. Answer: D

Explanation: Cooling equalizes temperatures, preventing bacterial growth and protein degradation. Warm-to-cold addition compromises safety and quality; prolonged storage before mixing violates hygiene protocols.

Q454. Answer: A

Explanation: Lower pressure relieves vascular constriction and pain. Frequency or topical care don't resolve mechanical misfit. Realignment ensures even suction and prevents tissue trauma.

Q455. Answer: A

Explanation: Gradual reduction allows hormonal equilibrium, avoiding engorgement or blocked ducts. Abrupt stopping causes discomfort. Oversupply regulation safeguards donor health and supply stability.

Q456. Answer: A

Explanation: SNS maintains nipple stimulation and infant coordination while providing extra milk. Bottles or pacifiers disrupt rhythm; spoon use is for short-term support only.

Q457. Answer: D

Explanation: Regular thorough washing removes residue and prevents bacterial colonization. Cold rinse or infrequent cleaning promotes microbial growth; sealed damp drying fosters contamination.

Q458. Answer: A

Explanation: Mimicking natural rhythms maintains hormonal cues and steady output. Skipping or consolidating sessions disrupts prolactin cycles, leading to gradual supply reduction and discomfort.

Q459. Answer: A

Explanation: Block methods reduce stimulation while relieving fullness safely. Over-pumping increases production; complete cessation risks engorgement. Alternating moderation balances comfort and control.

Q460. Answer: A

Explanation: Emotional well-being maintains sustainability and hormonal stability. Comparison or overexertion heightens stress and supply fluctuation. Compassionate counseling prevents burnout in exclusive expressers.

Q461. Answer: D

Explanation. Combining tactile bonding and mental health referral integrates psychosocial and physiological recovery. Emotional neglect worsens both lactation and attachment outcomes, while delayed feeding risks supply loss.

Q462. Answer: A

Explanation: Inclusive family participation promotes empathy and shared responsibility without reducing breastfeeding exclusivity. Formula substitution and avoidance isolate partners, compromising relational support.

Q463. Answer: A

Explanation: Psychological stress elevates muscle tone, intensifying perceived pain despite correct technique. Addressing relaxation and posture alleviates discomfort. Mechanical factors come secondary once emotional causes are considered.

Q464. Answer: A

Explanation: Positive reinforcement builds confidence and persistence critical in relactation. Comparison and unrealistic goals foster failure perception. Gradual stimulation reestablishes flow effectively with emotional resilience.

Q465. Answer: C

Explanation: Upright or reclined feeding slows milk flow and reduces reflux episodes. Supine positioning worsens symptoms. Proper angling balances gravity and comfort for controlled swallowing.

Q466. Answer: A

Explanation: Validation and practical coping empower confidence while preserving autonomy. Avoidance reinforces shame; substituting formula or denial undermines self-assurance and community normalization.

Q467. Answer: A

Explanation: Integrating technical and psychosocial strategies sustains supply while addressing mental fatigue. Quick pharmacologic fixes neglect root causes; empathy and structure restore hormonal balance.

Q468. Answer: A

Explanation: Trauma-informed care upholds autonomy and emotional safety, fostering trust and gradual participation. Physical insistence retraumatizes; sensitive adaptation preserves therapeutic relationship integrity.

Q469. Answer: D

Explanation: Assessing technical and emotional factors ensures equitable attention and confidence. Comparison undermines morale; balanced approach maintains milk flow and twin bonding quality.

Q470. Answer: A

Explanation: Respectful, evidence-based education replaces myth with understanding and preserves family harmony. Dismissive or impersonal communication damages rapport and acceptance.

Q471. Answer: A

Explanation: Empathetic affirmation rebuilds positive self-view linking nurturing capacity with strength. Technical diversion invalidates emotions, whereas acknowledgment supports long-term confidence and adherence.

Q472. Answer: A

Explanation: Gentle exposure rebuilds trust and reactivates instinctive reflexes disrupted by medical separation. Force or neglect causes aversion. Gradual reconditioning restores natural feeding behavior.

Q473. Answer: C

Explanation: Balanced documentation reduces stress while maintaining awareness. Over-monitoring increases anxiety, while no records may heighten uncertainty. Simplification preserves connection and confidence.

Q474. Answer: A

Explanation: Explicit consent ensures dignity and cross-cultural sensitivity. Physical intrusion or correction without context breaches trust. Interpreted dialogue maintains inclusivity and comprehension.

Q475. Answer: A

Explanation: Balanced reinforcement preserves morale and learning receptivity. Sole correction increases anxiety. Gentle, supportive feedback ensures retention and confidence in skill refinement.

Q476. Answer: A

Explanation: Validation alleviates guilt, preserving self-efficacy and ongoing breastfeeding interest. Rigid correction or avoidance undermines progress. Balanced education sustains trust and emotional recovery.

Q477. Answer: D

Explanation: Holistic care connects emotional treatment and lactation management for full recovery. Isolated or informal support lacks clinical structure, risking chronic stress and decreased breastfeeding success.

Q478. Answer: A

Explanation: Educating partners promotes shared understanding, reducing tension and supporting maternal confidence. Premature supplementation or avoidance weakens family unity and disrupts lactation rhythm.

Q479. Answer: A

Explanation: Combining physical demonstration and reassurance facilitates learning and emotional connection. Silence or detachment erodes motivation; written material alone cannot replace experiential practice.

Q480. Answer: A

Explanation: Compassionate flexibility supports healing and preserves supply without undue pressure. Emotional suppression or rigid control increases stress and physical risk. Sensitivity ensures humane, sustainable care.

Q481. Answer: B

Explanation: Poor latch leads to clicking sounds and nipple pain as suction breaks occur. The baby's chin should contact the breast for deep attachment. Rapid letdown may cause coughing, not clicking. Flat nipples alone don't cause audible sounds. Oversupply can exacerbate flow but not poor seal mechanics.

Q482. Answer: C

Explanation: Deep latch correction improves transfer efficiency, reducing fatigue and feeding time. Early repositioning prevents nipple trauma. Nipple shields or supplementation are secondary measures once technique fails. Extending feeding intervals worsens supply-demand feedback, potentially lowering milk production further.

Q483. Answer: C

Explanation: Weighing before and after feeding offers a direct quantitative measure of milk intake, reflecting effective transfer. Observation assesses behavior, not volume. It doesn't evaluate milk onset timing (lactogenesis II). This method ensures objective feedback for technique validation during clinical sessions.

Q484. Answer: B

Explanation: Effective hand expression uses gentle compressions behind the areola in a rhythmic pattern, mimicking suckling. Pulling or squeezing nipple tips can cause trauma. Pressure should not be at the nipple itself but along milk sinuses where oxytocin response facilitates flow.

Q485. Answer: A

Explanation: Side-lying or football holds reduce abdominal pressure and support recovery comfort while maintaining close contact. Upright cradle may strain incision. Prone or standing positions are unsafe for stability and latch. Position choice balances incision protection with optimal alignment for feeding.

Q486. Answer: A

Explanation: Refrigeration at 4°C preserves expressed milk safely for up to 24 hours. Warmer environments increase bacterial risk; freezing (0°C) is unnecessary for short-term storage. Maintaining hygiene during collection and labeling ensures consistency with NICU feeding protocols and safety standards.

Q487. Answer: A

Explanation: Excessive suction often causes edema and soreness; reducing vacuum prevents tissue injury. Correct flange sizing is essential but suction moderation comes first. Longer pumping worsens irritation. Warm compress aids comfort but doesn't address the mechanical cause directly.

Q488. Answer: C

Explanation: Audible swallowing and relaxation signify successful milk transfer and satiety. Persistent engorgement or drowsiness may indicate inefficient feeding. Maternal perception of fullness alone is unreliable. Observable feeding cues remain the most valid bedside indicators of adequacy.

Q489. Answer: A

Explanation: Vasospasm, often from shallow latch or cold exposure, causes post-feed blanching and sharp pain. Ensuring deeper latch reduces compression. Rapid letdown affects infant coordination, not maternal circulation. Blocked ducts or infection yield localized swelling or erythema, not blanching.

Q490. Answer: C

Explanation: The newborn's nutritional and immunological needs take precedence; they should feed first to ensure adequate intake. Alternating breasts can help manage supply but is secondary. Limiting sessions undermines bonding and production stability, counterproductive to tandem support principles.

Q491. Answer: B

Explanation: Poor arousal and ineffective latch often stem from suboptimal positioning and missed early cues. Evaluating readiness ensures improved transfer. Diet or anatomy alone rarely cause early fatigue. Behavioral observation and gentle stimulation optimize milk intake and energy balance.

Q492. Answer: B

Explanation: Vasospasm presents as burning or whitening of the nipple following feeding, often triggered by compression or cold. Candida causes shiny erythema, not blanching. Pump trauma localizes differently. Gentle heat and improved latch usually resolve symptoms.

Q493. Answer: B

Explanation: Breast compression helps sustain flow and milk ejection during sluggish feeding. It's effective for sleepy or weak infants. It's not primarily for engorgement or sensitivity. Combining compression with deep latch improves efficiency.

Q494. Answer: A

Explanation: Persistent firmness indicates poor milk drainage, often due to shallow latch or weak infant suction. Overproduction shows fullness pre-feed but softening post-feed. Early correction of technique prevents supply reduction and discomfort.

Q495. Answer: A

Explanation: Reclined positioning counters forceful letdown by reducing flow velocity. It allows gravity to modulate milk pace. Full pumping pre-feed depletes supply regulation, while shields are secondary options if posture fails.

Q496. Answer: A

Explanation: Nutritive sucking includes audible swallows and regular pauses indicating milk flow. Non-nutritive phases involve comfort suckling without swallow sounds. Recognizing these helps monitor effective feeding and infant satisfaction levels.

Q497. Answer: A

Explanation: Secure chin contact improves latch stability and prevents loss of suction. Mechanical or cosmetic interventions don't address underlying technique. Proper positioning ensures seal integrity and consistent feeding rhythm.

Q498. Answer: D

Explanation: Relaxation and visualization trigger oxytocin, enhancing milk ejection. Stress and mechanical overuse suppress reflex efficiency. Incorporating sensory cues promotes smoother, more productive sessions and emotional bonding.

Q499. Answer: A

Explanation: Asymmetrical latch techniques and breast shaping accommodate chin anatomy to achieve deeper attachment. Shields may be secondary aids. Posture alone doesn't solve mechanical depth issues critical to transfer.

Q500. Answer: A

Explanation: Comprehensive, accurate transfer documentation maintains care quality and protects safety. Verbal-only or client-mediated communication risks loss of details. Ethical professionalism includes continuity across caregivers.

Questions (501-600)

Q501. A consultant teaching a new mother about feeding cues emphasizes early signs of hunger. Which behavior should she highlight?

A. Crying loudly

B. Rooting and hand-to-mouth movement

C. Turning away from breast

D. Falling asleep

Q502. During a prenatal breastfeeding class, an IBCLC wants to maximize adult learning engagement. What is the most effective approach?

A. Provide long lectures with slides

B. Use interactive discussions and demonstrations

C. Assign textbook reading only

D. Focus solely on theoretical background

Q503. A consultant teaching a group of nurses about milk expression should emphasize which educational principle?

A. Adults learn best through repetition and memorization

B. Teaching should occur without demonstration

C. Facts alone are sufficient for retention

D. Learners need to connect content with practice

Q504. An IBCLC addresses a parent's anxiety about milk sufficiency. Which communication strategy is most effective?

A. Correct the parent's misconceptions immediately

B. Offer reassurance and normalize her experience

C. Provide lengthy technical explanations

D. Reassure without assessment

Q505. A client expresses guilt about supplementing with formula. How should the IBCLC respond?

A. Explain that formula is harmful

B. Reinforce parental choice and reframe success positively

C. Advise stopping formula immediately

D. Minimize her feelings

Q506. A mother confides that she feels inadequate compared to other parents online. What is the best IBCLC response?

A. Ignore social media discussion

B. Offer reassurance and normalize her experience

C. Advise quitting social media entirely

D. Emphasize online misinformation only

Q507. When documenting a consultation, what principle of professional record-keeping must be followed?

A. Include personal opinions about the client

B. Record objective findings and client statements

C. Summarize without time/date

D. Omit follow-up plans

Q508. A hospital IBCLC must obtain consent to share a mother's pumping data with neonatology. What legal principle applies?

A. Autonomy and confidentiality

B. Beneficence only

C. Justice

D. Nonmaleficence only

Q509. A consultant suspects another staff member is violating the WHO Code by promoting infant formula samples. What should she do first?

A. Ignore unless harm occurs
B. Report through institutional compliance channels
C. Confront the colleague publicly
D. Contact the formula company directly

Q510. A consultant counsels a working mother preparing to return to employment. Which recommendation aligns with best practice?

A. Pump only once daily
B. Begin pumping 2–3 weeks before return
C. Stop breastfeeding abruptly
D. Wait until after return to introduce bottle

Q511. An IBCLC designs an in-service session for pediatric staff. What educational strategy best improves retention?

A. Case-based problem solving
B. Memorization drills
C. Passive slide review
D. Reading assignments only

Q512. A mother hesitates to breastfeed in public. What supportive communication technique should the consultant use?

A. Normalize experience and explore comfort options
B. Discourage public feeding
C. Provide only written material
D. Avoid the topic

Q513. A parent appears overwhelmed during education. What adjustment should the IBCLC make?

A. Simplify and pace information delivery
B. Continue presenting full details
C. End session abruptly
D. Assign reading without discussion

Q514. A bilingual client struggles understanding instructions. What should the IBCLC do?

A. Skip education due to barrier
B. Ask family member to translate medical content
C. Simplify vocabulary only
D. Use certified interpreter services

Q515. A consultant receives feedback that her educational materials lack inclusivity. What is the best response?

A. Revise visuals and language to reflect diversity
B. Dismiss the feedback as opinion
C. Delay changes indefinitely
D. Focus only on text readability

Q516. Which approach builds trust when discussing sensitive topics like low supply?

A. Use empathetic tone and solution-focused language
B. Present data bluntly
C. Offer unsolicited personal anecdotes
D. Avoid the topic

Q517. A postpartum parent begins crying during a consult. What should the IBCLC do first?

A. Acknowledge emotion and pause to listen

B. Continue education uninterrupted
C. Leave the room immediately
D. Change topic

Q518. A consultant observes poor comprehension despite repeated explanation. What learning principle applies?
A. Stop education
B. Repeat same information louder
C. Shift topic
D. Vary teaching method and medium

Q519. What element most improves group education retention?
A. Interactive discussion and feedback loops
B. Sole lecture format
C. Dense handouts
D. Complex jargon

Q520. A consultant facilitates a team debrief after a challenging case. What is her main communication objective?
A. Encourage reflective learning and collective improvement
B. Assign blame for errors
C. Avoid feedback discussion
D. Limit conversation to senior staff

Q521. A consultant reviews a new study on exclusive breastfeeding rates. What is the first step in appraising its quality?
A. Identify the sample size and study design
B. Read the discussion only
C. Check author credentials only
D. Review funding source alone

Q522. A study shows a significant difference in milk composition after maternal exercise. What should the IBCLC check before applying findings to clients?
A. If it was widely shared on social media
B. If it aligns with personal belief
C. Whether peer review occurred and population relevance
D. Whether it was published in a local newsletter

Q523. When integrating research into clinical care, which step ensures ethical application?
A. Apply findings immediately to all clients
B. Evaluate client individuality and consent
C. Ignore data that contradicts experience
D. Use only old, established studies

Q524. A consultant compares two randomized controlled trials (RCTs) on nipple pain interventions. What makes RCTs valuable in lactation research?
A. They control bias through randomization
B. They are always inexpensive and quick
C. They avoid need for participant consent
D. They eliminate all confounding variables

Q525. An IBCLC designing a quality improvement project on hand expression success rates should first:
A. Define measurable outcomes and baseline data
B. Begin education sessions immediately
C. Collect testimonials
D. Skip institutional review

Q526. Which research source provides the most reliable breastfeeding data?
A. Peer-reviewed journal article
B. Personal blog post
C. Product marketing brochure
D. Social media influencer content
Q527. When interpreting statistical significance, what must the IBCLC also consider before drawing conclusions?
A. Funding organization
B. Author reputation
C. Whether results support popular opinion
D. Clinical relevance and effect size
Q528. A consultant reads a study stating, "Breastfeeding support groups increase duration." To assess credibility, she should first look at:
A. Study sample characteristics
B. Discussion section
C. References list
D. Conclusion summary
Q529. Which best describes evidence-based practice (EBP) in lactation consulting?
A. Integrating research, expertise, and client preference
B. Following only published protocols
C. Using intuition without data
D. Relying solely on past experience
Q530. What ethical safeguard must precede participant recruitment in lactation research?
A. Institutional Review Board (IRB) approval
B. Peer approval from colleagues
C. Verbal discussion with one participant
D. Publication agreement
Q531. A consultant uses recent Cochrane reviews to update policies. Why are systematic reviews valuable?
A. They present anecdotal evidence
B. They rely on expert opinion alone
C. They skip quality appraisal
D. They synthesize multiple studies for broader evidence
Q532. When reading a correlation study linking maternal caffeine intake and infant irritability, what key limitation must be remembered?
A. Correlation does not prove causation
B. Correlation always equals causation
C. Small samples guarantee accuracy
D. It is stronger than RCT evidence
Q533. An IBCLC reviewing community lactation outcomes notices conflicting studies. What is the best action?
A. Evaluate study design and consistency
B. Disregard all data
C. Choose the study that aligns personally
D. Assume both are wrong
Q534. Which factor most improves the reliability of breastfeeding research?
A. Large, diverse sample population
B. High author prestige

C. Short study duration
D. Anecdotal outcomes

Q535. A new meta-analysis suggests skin-to-skin contact reduces postpartum depression. What should the IBCLC prioritize before recommending practice changes?
A. Focus on author affiliations
B. Adopt change immediately
C. Ignore findings if not local
D. Assess study inclusion criteria and context

Q536. When applying evidence to diverse populations, what should IBCLCs always consider?
A. Cultural context and health disparities
B. Uniform global application
C. Language neutrality
D. Ignoring socioeconomic factors

Q537. An IBCLC presenting outcomes data should ensure which reporting element for credibility?
A. Transparency of limitations
B. Elimination of all bias statements
C. Overemphasis on positive results
D. Exclusion of failed data

Q538. A consultant evaluates a new herbal galactagogue study lacking control groups. What design limitation is evident?
A. Absence of comparison weakens validity
B. Enhanced generalizability
C. Complete elimination of bias
D. Guaranteed reliability

Q539. When using online research databases, which search strategy is most efficient for lactation evidence?
A. Avoid advanced search features
B. Use one-word search only
C. Search randomly without filters
D. Combine key terms with Boolean operators

Q540. A consultant summarizing study outcomes for colleagues must avoid which error?
A. Overgeneralizing beyond study parameters
B. Including key limitations
C. Stating context clearly
D. Citing references accurately

Q541. A consultant advocates for the Baby-Friendly Hospital Initiative (BFHI). What is the primary purpose of this global program?
A. Increase formula marketing access
B. Support evidence-based maternity care for breastfeeding
C. Promote rapid discharge after delivery
D. Reduce hospital staffing needs

Q542. When collaborating with local policymakers, what should an IBCLC prioritize to advocate effectively for breastfeeding programs?
A. Present emotional testimonials only
B. Provide data-driven evidence and community needs
C. Focus on hospital profitability
D. Avoid engagement with officials

Q543. A community initiative seeks to improve breastfeeding rates among low-income families. Which intervention reflects public health best practice?
A. Exclusive online materials
B. Peer counseling programs
C. Restrictive clinic scheduling
D. Free formula samples
Q544. An IBCLC presenting at a local health fair should focus messaging primarily on:
A. Technical clinical details
B. Simple, inclusive breastfeeding benefits
C. Institutional policies
D. Historical feeding trends
Q545. During an emergency shelter response, which breastfeeding support action aligns with WHO recommendations?
A. Encourage safe continued breastfeeding
B. Distribute infant formula broadly
C. Advise mothers to stop nursing temporarily
D. Separate infants from mothers for hygiene
Q546. A hospital seeks IBCLC input on compliance with the WHO Code. Which action best demonstrates adherence?
A. Removing promotional formula materials
B. Partnering with formula representatives for education
C. Displaying branded bottle posters
D. Offering coupons to new mothers
Q547. A public health nurse requests IBCLC guidance to design a breastfeeding awareness campaign. What should be emphasized?
A. Cultural sensitivity and local relevance
B. International imagery only
C. Complex medical terminology
D. Celebrity endorsements
Q548. What is the primary public health outcome linked to exclusive breastfeeding for six months?
A. Reduced maternal stress only
B. Lower infant morbidity and mortality
C. Increased healthcare costs
D. Decreased maternal bone density
Q549. An IBCLC attending a global conference advocates equitable lactation access. Which key principle aligns with social justice in public health?
A. Addressing systemic barriers to breastfeeding
B. Prioritizing urban populations only
C. Ignoring socioeconomic disparities
D. Promoting formula access equally
Q550. A consultant designs training for healthcare teams on BFHI Step 10 (Community support). Which key concept applies?
A. Strengthen post-discharge follow-up systems
B. Focus only on hospital discharge paperwork
C. Reduce referrals to external providers
D. Avoid community partnerships
Q551. A national survey reveals declining breastfeeding initiation rates. What policy-level strategy should IBCLCs advocate?

A. Paid maternity leave and workplace lactation rights
B. Mandatory weaning at 3 months
C. Increased formula advertising
D. Elimination of public breastfeeding areas

Q552. When supporting refugee populations, which IBCLC intervention aligns with cultural humility?
A. Enforce standard Western feeding plans
B. Begin instruction without questions
C. Assess feeding customs before advising
D. Discourage traditional foods

Q553. A regional coalition asks for IBCLC expertise on marketing ethics. Which guideline should she emphasize?
A. Transparency and avoidance of commercial bias
B. Promote specific brands for profit
C. Accept corporate sponsorship quietly
D. Focus only on social media popularity

Q554. An IBCLC working with adolescent mothers promotes peer mentor programs. What is the key advantage?
A. Age-aligned relatability and role modeling
B. Reduced need for professional consultants
C. Minimal engagement requirements
D. Focus on clinical interventions only

Q555. An IBCLC helps develop state breastfeeding report cards. What data should be prioritized?
A. Initiation, exclusivity, and duration rates
B. Hospital cafeteria menus
C. Marketing budgets
D. Maternal weight trends only

Q556. What is the most effective advocacy method for IBCLCs promoting hospital breastfeeding accreditation?
A. Ignore administrative feedback
B. Use emotional appeals only
C. Publicly shame non-compliant units
D. Present outcome data and patient stories

Q557. A consultant supports rural mothers lacking transport to clinics. Which public health partnership best addresses this barrier?
A. Telelactation services and mobile clinics
B. Limiting appointments to weekdays
C. Centralizing services in urban hospitals
D. Requiring in-person consults only

Q558. In global breastfeeding promotion, what is the role of IBCLCs?
A. Collaborate in policy development and education
B. Focus only on local clinic practice
C. Avoid political involvement
D. Limit advocacy to personal clients

Q559. Which communication element strengthens breastfeeding advocacy campaigns?
A. Consistent, culturally adapted messaging
B. Use of medical jargon for authority
C. Irregular message scheduling
D. Exclusive targeting of professionals

Q560. An IBCLC joins a multidisciplinary task force to support national breastfeeding goals. Which action aligns with collaborative advocacy?
A. Focus solely on clinical practice
B. Work independently from other members
C. Avoid data sharing
D. Contribute lactation expertise to policy recommendations
Q561. An IBCLC collaborates with pediatricians and dietitians for a preterm infant's discharge plan. What is her primary contribution?
A. Optimize feeding strategy for milk fortification and transition
B. Prescribe infant medications
C. Conduct developmental testing
D. Manage hospital budget
Q562. A multidisciplinary team develops postpartum care guidelines. How can the IBCLC best influence lactation integration?
A. Provide evidence-based recommendations during drafting
B. Wait until policies are finalized
C. Focus only on bedside teaching
D. Avoid interprofessional meetings
Q563. A consultant leads a training session for obstetric residents. What is the most effective educational objective?
A. Identify and correct common breastfeeding management errors
B. Memorize textbook definitions
C. Focus only on theory
D. Avoid role-play scenarios
Q564. A hospital's lactation program seeks Magnet® status accreditation. What performance measure should the IBCLC track?
A. Volunteer satisfaction surveys
B. Number of staff social events
C. Marketing material distribution
D. Exclusive breastfeeding rates at discharge
Q565. During a multidisciplinary meeting, the IBCLC identifies inconsistent documentation across units. What is her best advocacy step?
A. Propose standardized lactation charting templates
B. Criticize other staff publicly
C. Avoid raising concerns
D. Delegate documentation to volunteers
Q566. An IBCLC mentoring a new consultant emphasizes leadership competencies. Which trait should she model?
A. Accountability and reflective practice
B. Authoritarian decision-making
C. Minimal feedback to mentees
D. Avoidance of interprofessional input
Q567. A lactation service introduces outcome dashboards for quality improvement. Which metric is most meaningful for evaluating consultant impact?
A. Duration of exclusive breastfeeding at six weeks
B. Number of social media posts
C. Consultant attendance hours
D. Advertising reach

Q568. An IBCLC joins a research committee reviewing breastfeeding interventions. What role enhances her professional credibility?
A. Approve all projects without review
B. Decline involvement to avoid conflict
C. Focus solely on administrative duties
D. Provide subject expertise and critical appraisal of lactation studies
Q569. To sustain program funding, an IBCLC must present measurable outcomes. What type of data best supports her report?
A. Quantitative breastfeeding rate trends
B. Staff lunch attendance
C. Consultant anecdotes
D. Facility floor plans
Q570. A consultant leading a coalition proposes training community health workers. Which outcome represents leadership success?
A. Increased community breastfeeding initiation
B. Improved consultant salary structure
C. Higher product sales
D. Fewer follow-up visits
Q571. An IBCLC supervises interns in a teaching hospital. What supervision method ensures optimal competency development?
A. Direct observation with immediate feedback
B. Minimal oversight to foster independence
C. Delayed evaluation after program completion
D. Exclusive reliance on written exams
Q572. A lactation consultant developing educational policy for nurses should ensure what component?
A. Unstructured informal sessions
B. Optional participation
C. Random topic selection
D. Inclusion of standardized competency checklists
Q573. A consultant observes conflict between two team members regarding patient care. What leadership approach fosters resolution?
A. Facilitate open communication and mediation
B. Take sides immediately
C. Ignore the disagreement
D. Escalate to administration instantly
Q574. A hospital IBCLC designs a training initiative to meet Joint Commission perinatal standards. What should guide her program objectives?
A. National benchmarks and patient outcome data
B. Staff preferences only
C. Marketing recommendations
D. External vendor input
Q575. A consultant evaluating her leadership impact uses self-reflection tools. What is the main benefit?
A. Identifying personal growth areas and enhancing accountability
B. Eliminating need for peer feedback
C. Prioritizing personal comfort
D. Avoiding performance data
Q576. A lactation manager leads a quality committee. What is the committee's primary function?
A. Manage catering services

B. Approve staff vacation schedules
C. Develop retail promotions
D. Evaluate and improve breastfeeding care processes

Q577. A regional IBCLC coordinator implements a mentorship network. Which goal aligns with professional leadership development?

A. Build peer support and knowledge exchange
B. Replace certification exams
C. Limit membership participation
D. Focus solely on administrative issues

Q578. During a program audit, the IBCLC identifies data discrepancies. What is her ethical duty?

A. Report findings transparently for correction
B. Conceal errors to protect reputation
C. Alter records before review
D. Ignore unless discovered

Q579. A lactation consultant advocates for inclusion of breastfeeding metrics in national health databases. What is the key benefit?

A. Enhanced policy planning and funding allocation
B. Increased consultant workload
C. Reduced research transparency
D. Elimination of local programs

Q580. A consultant presenting lactation leadership outcomes to stakeholders should emphasize:

A. Personal challenges faced
B. Measurable improvements and strategic goals
C. Irrelevant anecdotes
D. Confidential data disclosure

Q581. An IBCLC encounters a cultural practice that includes supplementing newborns with herbal tea. What is her most appropriate response?

A. Respectfully explore the tradition and discuss evidence-based risks
B. Condemn the practice immediately
C. Report the family to authorities
D. Ignore the information

Q582. A consultant is asked by a formula company to present at a conference with compensation. What should she do first?

A. Decline if it violates WHO Code and IBCLC ethics
B. Accept to promote professional exposure
C. Request additional payment
D. Present product marketing slides

Q583. During documentation review, an IBCLC notices missing informed consent for a research participant. What is her ethical obligation?

A. Pause study activity and report to supervisor
B. Continue the study quietly
C. Alter documentation retroactively
D. Disregard oversight

Q584. When developing a multidisciplinary policy on infant feeding, which element ensures legal compliance?

A. Historical norms
B. Institutional preference alone
C. Marketing input from industry

D. Alignment with national breastfeeding legislation and WHO Code

Q585. A consultant providing virtual care notices a mother filming sessions without consent. What should she do?

A. Reiterate confidentiality and request stopping the recording
B. Ignore to maintain rapport
C. End call immediately without explanation
D. Record the session herself

Q586. An IBCLC preparing community materials includes diverse family images. Why is this important?

A. Promotes inclusivity and cultural representation
B. Meets marketing requirements
C. Reduces cost
D. Increases technical complexity

Q587. A client discloses domestic violence during a consultation. What should the IBCLC do next?

A. Ensure safety, follow mandated reporting protocols, and refer appropriately
B. Ignore to maintain focus on feeding
C. Offer personal counseling beyond scope
D. Document but avoid follow-up

Q588. A consultant supervising students must evaluate performance fairly. What method best supports ethical assessment?

A. Use arbitrary comparison
B. Grade based on personal rapport
C. Adjust scores to avoid complaints
D. Use transparent, criterion-based evaluation tools

Q589. When discussing human milk donation, which ethical issue is most critical?

A. Informed consent and screening transparency
B. Financial compensation negotiation
C. Religious endorsement
D. Supply marketing

Q590. A consultant develops social media content for her practice. What must she ensure?

A. Maintain professional boundaries and evidence-based accuracy
B. Share client photos freely
C. Prioritize engagement over accuracy
D. Post personal opinions as clinical advice

Q591. A hospital ethics committee asks for IBCLC input on feeding decisions for an infant with life-limiting illness. What is her role?

A. Provide expertise on lactation and family-centered feeding options
B. Decide care independently
C. Decline participation
D. Offer nonclinical opinions

Q592. When counseling a mother living with HIV in a country supporting safe formula use, the IBCLC should:

A. Provide advice based on personal belief
B. Recommend exclusive breastfeeding globally
C. Discourage all formula feeding
D. Follow national guidelines and support informed choice

Q593. A consultant finds her colleague documenting client data in unsecured notes. What is the ethical response?

A. Address confidentiality breach and report per policy

B. Ignore unless discovered
C. Delete notes without consent
D. Discuss casually with others

Q594. An IBCLC chairing a professional association drafts new practice standards. What key element ensures credibility?
A. Transparent consensus with stakeholder input
B. Exclusive internal decision-making
C. Marketing-based development
D. Limited peer review

Q595. A consultant receives a client gift after discharge. What is the ethical approach?
A. Graciously decline gifts of monetary value
B. Accept all tokens to maintain rapport
C. Publicly display gifts on social media
D. Exchange for professional discounts

Q596. An IBCLC writing a research article must avoid which ethical breach?
A. Peer review participation
B. Accurate citation of sources
C. Disclosure of funding
D. Plagiarism or duplicate publication

Q597. When teaching healthcare students, how should the IBCLC model professionalism?
A. Demonstrate evidence-based empathy and accountability
B. Share personal frustrations
C. Use hierarchical control
D. Avoid emotional engagement

Q598. A consultant discovers a local group promoting unsafe feeding practices. What is her professional responsibility?
A. Provide corrective education using current evidence
B. Publicly shame the group
C. Ignore misinformation
D. Engage in online arguments

Q599. An IBCLC developing mentorship programs for rural practitioners should focus on:
A. Prioritizing administrative tasks
B. Limiting mentor contact
C. Building remote peer networks and continuing education
D. Excluding non-clinical support

Q600. A senior IBCLC concludes a leadership presentation with global colleagues. Which statement best summarizes professional commitment?
A. Upholding ethics, evidence, and equity in lactation care
B. Expanding personal brand reach
C. Prioritizing competition among consultants
D. Reducing transparency in policy work

Answer key and Explanation (501-600)

Q501. Answer: B

Explanation: Early cues such as rooting, lip smacking, and hand-to-mouth movements signal readiness before distress. Crying is a late cue leading to poor latch. Turning away suggests fatigue, not hunger. Recognizing subtle behaviors promotes calmer, more effective feeding sessions and supports bonding.

Q502. Answer: B

Explanation: Interactive teaching using role-play, models, and discussion enhances retention by appealing to adult learners' experience-based motivation. Lectures or readings alone reduce engagement. Combining theory with demonstration bridges knowledge and practice, aligning with adult learning principles in lactation education.

Q503. Answer: D

Explanation: Adult learners integrate knowledge effectively when linked to real scenarios. Practical demonstrations on pump use reinforce conceptual understanding. Memorization or fact delivery without context leads to poor application. Linking to workplace experience improves competency and confidence in supporting mothers.

Q504. Answer: B

Explanation: Using open-ended questions encourages sharing and helps explore underlying fears. Reflective listening builds trust, allowing tailored education. Immediate correction or excessive information may heighten anxiety. Empathic communication fosters confidence and strengthens consultant–parent rapport during sensitive discussions.

Q505. Answer: B

Explanation: Validating emotion and affirming the parent's efforts promotes empowerment. Positive reframing supports continued breastfeeding and emotional well-being. Negative judgment or abrupt cessation creates guilt and noncompliance. The consultant balances empathy with evidence-based encouragement for partial or exclusive breastfeeding goals.

Q506. Answer: B

Explanation: Validating emotions and normalizing struggles reduces comparison stress. Reassurance that variations in experience are normal supports resilience. Advising social withdrawal or focusing solely on misinformation may feel dismissive. Compassionate acknowledgment restores confidence in her unique breastfeeding journey.

Q507. Answer: B

Explanation: Accurate, objective documentation ensures continuity, legal integrity, and ethical compliance. Client statements should be quoted; professional impressions clearly labeled. Subjective remarks or missing timelines compromise records. Proper charting supports multidisciplinary collaboration and protects both practitioner and client.

Q508. Answer: A

Explanation: Autonomy grants clients control over personal data, and confidentiality mandates explicit consent before sharing. Even beneficial intentions require informed permission. Upholding these principles reinforces ethical conduct and institutional compliance with patient privacy laws in lactation care.

Q509. Answer: B

Explanation: Reporting through established compliance or ethics procedures maintains professionalism and accountability. Public confrontation risks conflict, while direct contact with companies breaches protocol. Following chain-of-command ensures advocacy aligns with institutional and global ethical standards like the WHO Code.

Q510. Answer: B

Explanation: Gradual pumping introduction before work transition helps build supply and familiarize the infant with expressed milk. Abrupt weaning or delayed bottle practice increases stress. Consistent pumping schedules sustain lactation while balancing occupational responsibilities and maternal comfort.

Q511. Answer: A

Explanation: Case-based learning reinforces understanding through contextual decision-making. It increases engagement and application. Memorization or passive methods lack experiential depth needed in clinical lactation settings.

Q512. Answer: A

Explanation: Normalization reduces stigma, while offering strategies like nursing covers builds confidence. Avoidance or discouragement undermines maternal empowerment and rights.

Q513. Answer: A

Explanation: Tailoring pacing supports comprehension and retention. Overloading information impairs learning, especially postpartum. Gentle pacing fosters reassurance and engagement.

Q514. Answer: D

Explanation: Certified interpreters ensure accuracy and confidentiality. Family translators may distort meaning. Simplification helps but cannot replace precise communication essential to clinical care.

Q515. Answer: A

Explanation: Inclusive materials promote belonging and accessibility. Proactive revision demonstrates responsiveness and professionalism. Ignoring feedback risks alienation and reduces impact.

Q516. Answer: A

Explanation: Empathy and solution framing sustain morale and openness. Harsh or impersonal communication discourages dialogue. Compassionate delivery reinforces therapeutic relationships and adherence.

Q517. Answer: A

Explanation: Emotional validation strengthens rapport and allows recovery. Ignoring distress creates disengagement. Listening provides space for empathy, facilitating holistic support.

Q518. Answer: D

Explanation: Adults have diverse learning styles; incorporating visual, auditory, and hands-on aids improves understanding. Repetition alone fails if the approach doesn't match the learner's mode.

Q519. Answer: A

Explanation: Engagement and feedback foster active learning. Monologues or excessive jargon reduce retention. Group dialogue empowers participants and reinforces mutual learning.

Q520. Answer: A

Explanation: Reflective debriefing transforms experiences into learning opportunities and promotes non-punitive culture. Blame inhibits growth. Inclusive dialogue supports teamwork and emotional resilience.

Q521. Answer: A

Explanation: Assessing methodology—especially design and sample size—determines validity and generalizability. Author identity or funding adds context but doesn't define reliability. Critical appraisal begins with understanding how evidence was generated and whether its findings apply to clinical lactation populations.

Q522. Answer: C

Explanation: Peer review confirms methodological rigor, while population matching ensures appropriate translation to practice. Personal or social approval lacks scientific basis. Reliable implementation requires verified data quality and contextual fit within maternal physiology and breastfeeding science.

Q523. Answer: B

Explanation: Ethical evidence-based care respects autonomy and diversity, applying findings selectively with consent. Blind adoption risks inappropriate use. Outdated studies may not reflect current standards. Client-centered application ensures safety and promotes trust in lactation evidence translation.

Q524. Answer: A

Explanation: Randomization reduces selection bias, strengthening internal validity. While not flawless, RCTs represent gold-standard designs for evaluating interventions. Cost and ethics still apply, but systematic control distinguishes RCTs as cornerstone methodology in breastfeeding evidence hierarchies.

Q525. Answer: A

Explanation: Establishing measurable, baseline outcomes supports evaluation and ethical oversight. Education or testimonials lack quantifiable rigor. Institutional approval ensures accountability. Data definition aligns project intent with improvement goals and clinical quality assurance requirements.

Q526. Answer: A

Explanation: Peer-reviewed articles undergo expert scrutiny for validity and accuracy. Informal media may include bias or unsupported claims. Lactation consultants rely on credible sources to guide professional practice and protect families from misinformation or commercial influence.

Q527. Answer: D

Explanation: Significant p-values alone may lack practical importance; evaluating effect size and clinical relevance ensures real-world applicability. Research translation demands critical thinking beyond statistical symbols, focusing on meaningful outcomes for breastfeeding dyads.

Q528. Answer: A

Explanation: Reviewing participant demographics determines generalizability to local populations. If samples differ markedly, applicability weakens. The discussion and conclusion interpret findings, but understanding who was studied is essential to context-based lactation practice.

Q529. Answer: A

Explanation: EBP merges scientific evidence, professional skill, and client values for balanced, individualized care. Exclusive reliance on protocols or intuition neglects dynamic decision-making. IBCLCs apply integrated reasoning to optimize outcomes while maintaining evidence alignment.

Q530. Answer: A

Explanation: IRB oversight ensures participant protection, informed consent, and compliance with research ethics. Colleague input or publication plans cannot replace formal review. In breastfeeding research, vulnerable populations require strict adherence to regulatory standards.

Q531. Answer: D

Explanation: Systematic reviews aggregate and evaluate existing research, reducing bias and enhancing generalizability. Unlike expert commentary, they follow structured inclusion criteria and rigorous appraisal, offering IBCLCs consolidated evidence for guideline formulation.

Q532. Answer: A

Explanation: Correlation identifies relationships but not direct cause-effect. Confounding factors may influence observed links. Understanding this prevents misinterpretation when advising clients about caffeine and infant behavior, maintaining evidence-based and responsible guidance.

Q533. Answer: A

Explanation: Comparing design, sample, and context helps identify sources of discrepancy and determine reliability. Discarding or selecting data by bias undermines credibility. Systematic evaluation supports nuanced, professional judgment in evidence interpretation.

Q534. Answer: A

Explanation: Larger, diverse samples enhance external validity, ensuring findings reflect broader populations. Prestige or brevity doesn't ensure accuracy. Representative sampling supports inclusivity and cultural applicability, critical for global lactation care consistency.

Q535. Answer: D

Explanation: Evaluating inclusion criteria ensures data comparability and contextual validity. Immediate adoption risks misapplication. Evidence integration requires critical appraisal to align with maternal care environments and individual mental health needs.

Q536. Answer: A

Explanation: Evidence must adapt to cultural, economic, and systemic realities to remain equitable. Ignoring disparities perpetuates inequity. Inclusive application ensures lactation support reflects diverse maternal experiences and community health determinants.

Q537. Answer: A

Explanation: Acknowledging study limitations fosters transparency and scientific honesty, essential for evidence-based credibility. Concealing or omitting data undermines trust. Balanced reporting advances professional integrity and encourages continual research improvement.

Q538. Answer: A

Explanation: Without control, causation cannot be confirmed; placebo or standard comparison strengthens reliability. Observational design limits interpretive power. IBCLCs interpret such studies cautiously, acknowledging confounding factors before advising clients.

Q539. Answer: D

Explanation: Boolean logic (AND, OR, NOT) refines searches, ensuring relevance and efficiency. Strategic filtering enhances precision in finding current lactation studies, supporting efficient evidence retrieval and scholarly accuracy in IBCLC research practice.

Q540. Answer: A

Explanation: Overgeneralization distorts findings and misguides practice. Responsible summaries specify scope, sample, and context, preserving integrity. Accurate citation ensures reproducibility, crucial for collaborative, evidence-based lactation education.

Q541. Answer: B

Explanation: The BFHI encourages hospitals to implement Ten Steps promoting exclusive breastfeeding and maternal support. It standardizes evidence based maternity care, not marketing or discharge acceleration. Staff training and policy alignment foster global breastfeeding success and maternal–infant health outcomes.

Q542. Answer: B

Explanation: Policymakers respond best to evidence-based data highlighting population health benefits. Presenting measurable outcomes supports funding and policy creation. Emotional appeals alone lack sustainability, while avoiding engagement forfeits professional advocacy influence.

Q543. Answer: B

Explanation: Peer counseling provides accessible, culturally congruent support proven to improve breastfeeding duration in underserved populations. Free formula undermines breastfeeding rates. Accessibility and relational outreach define equitable, effective public health interventions.

Q544. Answer: B

Explanation: Public outreach should emphasize clear, inclusive education on breastfeeding's health, economic, and emotional benefits. Technical jargon alienates community audiences. Simplified, culturally respectful messaging strengthens awareness and motivation across diverse populations.

Q545. Answer: A

Explanation: In crises, breastfeeding remains safest due to sterile, readily available nutrition and immune protection. Formula use without sanitation increases infection risk. Maintaining proximity and feeding continuity supports infant survival and maternal stability.

Q546. Answer: A

Explanation: WHO Code compliance prohibits marketing materials and corporate promotion in healthcare settings. Removing branded advertising ensures ethical neutrality. Partnership or incentive programs undermine credibility and global public health commitments.

Q547. Answer: A

Explanation: Campaigns succeed when culturally tailored and community-informed. Understanding local norms increases acceptance and impact. Global or celebrity messages risk disconnect unless contextually integrated. IBCLCs ensure evidence-based, culturally respectful communication strategies.

Q548. Answer: B

Explanation: Exclusive breastfeeding significantly reduces infectious disease risk and mortality. It benefits both maternal and infant health, lowering system costs. Other options misrepresent physiological outcomes or financial implications of breastfeeding promotion.

Q549. Answer: A

Explanation: Advocacy grounded in equity seeks to dismantle systemic barriers—poverty, workplace policy, cultural bias—that hinder breastfeeding. Inclusive initiatives extend beyond urban focus. Promoting formula equivalence contradicts health equity principles and WHO standards.

Q550. Answer: A

Explanation: Step 10 stresses post-discharge continuity and community referral systems for sustained breastfeeding success. Collaboration with local organizations enhances maternal support networks. Limiting or avoiding partnerships contradicts BFHI standards and continuity principles.

Q551. Answer: A

Explanation: Policy support through paid leave and lactation accommodations enables sustained breastfeeding. Restrictive or anti-breastfeeding policies worsen disparities. Advocacy at legislative levels ensures structural empowerment for working parents.

Q552. Answer: C

Explanation: Cultural humility requires assessment before action. Understanding traditional feeding norms ensures respect and trust. Imposing standardized approaches or rejecting cultural foods alienates families and compromises support effectiveness.

Q553. Answer: A

Explanation: Ethical marketing upholds transparency, neutrality, and client welfare. Commercial influence undermines credibility and WHO Code compliance. IBCLCs maintain independence, advocating accurate, unbiased breastfeeding education.

Q554. Answer: A

Explanation: Peer mentorship fosters trust, relevance, and sustainable support among young mothers. Shared experience enhances confidence and breastfeeding duration. Professional oversight remains complementary, ensuring evidence-based alignment and program integrity.

Q555. Answer: A

Explanation: Key breastfeeding indicators measure initiation, exclusivity, and continuation—core metrics for public health progress. Ancillary data may inform context but lacks direct outcome value. These measures guide resource allocation and program evaluation.

Q556. Answer: D

Explanation: Combining outcome evidence with patient narratives strengthens persuasive advocacy. Balanced messaging appeals to both data-driven and empathetic stakeholders. Negative tactics or disregard for collaboration harm institutional relationships and professional reputation.

Q557. Answer: A

Explanation: Mobile and telehealth solutions improve accessibility for geographically isolated families. Restrictive scheduling or centralized services deepen inequity. Technology-enabled outreach aligns with inclusive, innovative lactation public health models.

Q558. Answer: A

Explanation: IBCLCs engage across clinical, policy, and educational levels to influence systemic breastfeeding support. Limiting advocacy scope reduces impact. Global collaboration enhances consistency with WHO, UNICEF, and professional lactation frameworks.

Q559. Answer: A

Explanation: Advocacy success depends on clear, culturally relevant communication sustained through consistent outreach. Technical language isolates audiences, and inconsistent scheduling weakens recall. Inclusion across demographics maximizes awareness and acceptance.

Q560. Answer: D

Explanation: Integrating lactation knowledge strengthens comprehensive maternal-child health strategies. Collaboration ensures breastfeeding considerations are embedded in broader policy frameworks. Isolation or withholding data undermines unified progress and interprofessional respect.

Q561. Answer: A

Explanation: The IBCLC ensures appropriate breast milk handling, fortification, and feeding methods to meet preterm nutritional needs. Medication or budgeting lies outside her scope. Collaboration with nutrition and neonatology integrates lactation into interdisciplinary discharge continuity.

Q562. Answer: A

Explanation: Early participation ensures lactation perspectives are embedded in policies. Waiting until finalization limits influence. IBCLCs advocate breastfeeding inclusion during planning, aligning maternal-child protocols with global best practices and institutional care standards.

Q563. Answer: A

Explanation: Interactive, case-based learning fosters critical thinking and clinical problem-solving. Memorization alone lacks application depth. Role-play and error correction reinforce skills essential for evidence-based interdisciplinary collaboration in lactation care.

Q564. Answer: D

Explanation: Exclusive breastfeeding at discharge reflects patient-centered quality and aligns with Magnet® nursing excellence metrics. Nonclinical metrics do not indicate lactation program success. Tracking outcomes demonstrates evidence-based nursing leadership impact.

Q565. Answer: A

Explanation: Consistent documentation enhances continuity, legal protection, and research reliability. Collaborative proposal of standardized tools promotes efficiency and reduces errors without assigning blame, fostering quality improvement and shared accountability.

Q566. Answer: A

Explanation: Effective leaders model accountability, self-reflection, and collaborative learning. Authoritarian styles hinder growth. Constructive feedback promotes professional development and mutual respect within multidisciplinary lactation teams.

Q567. Answer: A

Explanation: Exclusive breastfeeding duration demonstrates direct patient impact. Attendance or publicity metrics lack correlation with outcomes. Dashboards help visualize data-driven service improvement tied to maternal–infant health measures.

Q568. Answer: D

Explanation: Contributing specialized lactation insight and critical evaluation establishes authority and interdisciplinary respect. Nonparticipation forfeits influence. Ethical, evidence-based collaboration ensures methodological soundness in breastfeeding-related research.

Q569. Answer: A

Explanation: Quantitative data on breastfeeding rates provides objective evidence of program effectiveness. Anecdotes and unrelated metrics lack evaluative rigor. Data-driven reporting strengthens administrative and policy-level support.

Q570. Answer: A

Explanation: Leadership effectiveness manifests through measurable health outcomes, not personal gain. Improved community breastfeeding rates signify empowerment and systemic progress derived from capacity-building initiatives.

Q571. Answer: A

Explanation: Real-time supervision identifies skill gaps promptly, allowing correction and growth. Independence evolves gradually. Continuous formative feedback underpins experiential learning and confidence in clinical practice.

Q572. Answer: D

Explanation: Structured competency checklists ensure consistent assessment and skill validation. Optional or unstructured learning lacks accountability. Standardization supports quality assurance and professional readiness in lactation care training.

Q573. Answer: A

Explanation: Encouraging dialogue promotes mutual understanding and trust. Mediation resolves conflict constructively. Avoidance or bias intensifies tension. Effective leaders uphold collaboration and emotional intelligence within interprofessional teams.

Q574. Answer: A

Explanation: Alignment with benchmarks and outcomes ensures compliance and relevance. Personal or commercial influences compromise focus. Data-driven goals maintain quality alignment with recognized healthcare accreditation requirements.

Q575. Answer: A

Explanation: Self-assessment fosters continuous improvement and insight into strengths and limitations. Excluding feedback or data limits perspective. Reflective leaders demonstrate adaptability and evidence-informed decision-making.

Q576. Answer: D

Explanation: Quality committees analyze care systems to enhance effectiveness and outcomes. Administrative or unrelated duties are secondary. Evidence-based reviews drive institutional excellence and program accreditation.

Q577. Answer: A

Explanation: Mentorship strengthens community, builds confidence, and maintains standards through shared learning. Restrictive or administrative-only focus limits growth. Collaborative networks enhance sustainability and competence across regions.

Q578. Answer: A

Explanation: Ethical integrity demands honest disclosure and remediation. Concealment damages credibility and violates professional conduct. Transparency supports institutional trust and continuous improvement culture.

Q579. Answer: A

Explanation: National data integration informs health policy, resource distribution, and strategic breastfeeding promotion. Broader visibility enhances recognition of lactation outcomes as vital indicators of maternal–infant health.

Q580. Answer: B

Explanation: Presenting outcomes tied to measurable progress and strategic alignment demonstrates professionalism and accountability. Personal or confidential details distract from objective impact assessment essential to leadership reporting.

Q581. Answer: A

Explanation: Cultural sensitivity requires respectful inquiry and evidence-based discussion. Immediate condemnation damages rapport, while ignoring risks neglects care duty. Engaging collaboratively promotes informed decision-making within the family's cultural framework.

Q582. Answer: A

Explanation: Accepting sponsorship from formula companies breaches the WHO Code and IBCLC professional standards. Ethical consultants maintain independence to avoid conflicts of interest. Transparency and adherence to global ethics protect professional integrity.

Q583. Answer: A

Explanation: Missing consent violates participant rights and ethical standards. Halting procedures and notifying appropriate oversight maintains research integrity. Retroactive changes constitute misconduct and breach professional trust.

Q584. Answer: D

Explanation: Policies must align with legal and international frameworks protecting breastfeeding. Institutional habits or commercial influence lack legitimacy. Consistency with law and ethics safeguards patient rights and organizational accountability.

Q585. Answer: A

Explanation: Protecting privacy requires addressing consent respectfully. Explaining confidentiality standards educates clients while preserving professionalism. Abrupt termination or reciprocal recording breaches trust and ethics.

Q586. Answer: A

Explanation: Visual inclusivity validates varied family structures and cultural identities, promoting accessibility and equity in public education. Representation enhances connection and reduces stigma in breastfeeding promotion efforts.

Q587. Answer: A

Explanation: Ensuring client safety takes precedence. Following reporting laws and connecting with support services respects scope and duty of care. Providing unqualified counseling exceeds IBCLC practice boundaries.

Q588. Answer: D

Explanation: Objective, criterion-referenced evaluation ensures fairness and accountability in education. Bias or favoritism undermines credibility and student trust. Ethical assessment reinforces standards and learning integrity.

Q589. Answer: A

Explanation: Informed consent ensures donors understand screening, storage, and distribution. Transparency protects recipients and upholds donor rights. Commercial or ideological concerns are secondary to ethical safety and respect.

Q590. Answer: A

Explanation: Online professionalism demands privacy protection and factual accuracy. Sharing personal data or unverified advice breaches ethics. Evidence-based content builds credibility and public trust in lactation care.

Q591. Answer: A

Explanation: The IBCLC contributes evidence-informed insights on human milk benefits and emotional aspects while respecting family choices. Decision-making remains collaborative. Participation reflects ethical, interdisciplinary professionalism.

Q592. Answer: D

Explanation: Guidance must align with national HIV and infant feeding policies to ensure safety and cultural context. Personal opinion cannot override evidence or legal frameworks. Supporting informed, individualized decisions ensures ethical compliance.

Q593. Answer: A

Explanation: Protecting client confidentiality requires prompt reporting through institutional procedures. Ignoring or gossiping compounds risk. Proper documentation safeguards legal compliance and ethical accountability.

Q594. Answer: A

Explanation: Inclusive, transparent development invites diverse expertise, promoting legitimacy and adoption. Secretive or biased processes erode trust. Broad review guarantees accuracy and representation across the profession.

Q595. Answer: A

Explanation: Ethical guidelines discourage accepting valuable gifts to prevent conflict of interest. Acknowledging gratitude respectfully maintains professional boundaries. Public display or exchange compromises impartiality and trust.

Q596. Answer: D

Explanation: Plagiarism undermines scientific integrity and violates publication ethics. Proper citation and disclosure maintain transparency. Upholding authorship ethics preserves credibility and protects the lactation field's scholarly reputation.

Q597. Answer: A

Explanation: Modeling professionalism through empathy and responsibility sets a standard for compassionate, science-informed care. Negative or detached behavior discourages learning and teamwork. Ethical educators inspire excellence through integrity.

Q598. Answer: A

Explanation: Professional advocacy involves constructive correction through education. Confrontation or neglect perpetuates harm. Delivering accurate information diplomatically safeguards public health and professional credibility.

Q599. Answer: C

Explanation: Remote mentorship extends access, fosters peer learning, and sustains practice standards. Restricting engagement weakens professional growth. Inclusive support ensures equitable development opportunities across diverse practice settings.

Q600. Answer: A

Explanation: Ethical, equitable, evidence-based care defines IBCLC professionalism worldwide. Integrity and collaboration strengthen public trust and global maternal–infant health outcomes. Personal or competitive motives detract from collective professional advancement.

Made in United States
Orlando, FL
04 November 2026

90201052R00087